The Meaty Truth

The Meaty Truth

Why Our Food Is Destroying Our Health and Environment —and Who Is Responsible

Shushana Castle and Amy-Lee Goodman
Foreword by Dr. Neal Barnard

Skyhorse Publishing

Skyhorse Publishing books may be purchased in bulk at special discounts for sales promotion, corporate gifts, fund-raising, or educational purposes. Special editions can also be created to specifications. For details, contact the Special Sales Department, Skyhorse Publishing, 307 West 36th Street, 11th Floor, New York, NY 10018 or info@skyhorsepublishing.com.

Skyhorse® and Skyhorse Publishing® are registered trademarks of Skyhorse Publishing, Inc.®, a Delaware corporation.

Visit our website at www.skyhorsepublishing.com.

10 9 8 7 6 5 4 3 2 1

Library of Congress Cataloging-in-Publication Data is available on file.

Cover design by Owen Corrigan
Cover photo credit Thinkstock

Print ISBN: 978-1-62914-427-6
Ebook ISBN: 978-1-63220-044-0

Printed in the United States of America

Acknowledgments

First and foremost, this book would not have been possible without the passionate and fearless leaders in the health, environmental, and animal movements that opened our eyes and left us forever changed. We would not be who we are today without the pioneers who came before us—John Robbins, Dr. Neal Barnard, Dr. T. Colin Campbell, Gene Bauer, Francis Moore Lappe, and so many others we wish to mention. We are forever indebted to your hard work and dedication to improving the lives of all the animals and the health of our planet.

To those who shared their stories with us, especially Karen Hudson, Helen Reddout, Howard Lyman, and Robyn O'Brien—thank you for letting us publicize the ever-evolving stories in your communities. Your hard work demanding justice and healthier food is an inspiration to us all.

We are grateful to the experts who were instrumental in *The Meaty Truth's* publication. Our wonderful agent, Steve Harris, provided advice and guidance throughout the publishing process. Our illustrator, Julia O'Flynn O'Brien, made our cartoons come to life. Our editor, Emily Houlihan, publisher Bill Wolfsthal, and the entire Skyhorse team worked closely with us to share this untold story and expose the truth.

To our families and dear friends, your endless support, encouragement, and patience allowed us to pursue this dream and see it become a reality after many years of hard work. And finally to all the animals, domestic and wild, you fill our lives with so much joy and remind us each day why we wrote *The Meaty Truth*. Thank you.

Dedication

To Mom, Dad, Greg, and Jay, whose love and encouragement taught me to always dream big.

And to Mom and Jack, your love and support is bigger than the universe. Thank you.

Contents

Foreword

When I was growing up in Fargo, North Dakota, our family ate roast beef, baked potatoes, and corn. Day after day, that was about it. Sometimes a pork chop or slice of liver might replace the beef. But we never strayed very far from this rather unimaginative, meat-centered menu. After all, we thought we needed meat for iron and protein—which translated into health and strength—and we were prepared to overlook the unsavory aspects of slaughter and meat packing. Never mind that heart attacks were common—and still are. We attributed them to old age, or perhaps genetics, rather than to our meaty diet.

Later on, when I entered medical school, I learned something quite different. It turned out that people who avoided meat were healthier than those who ate it. Carefully conducted research studies showed that they were slimmer; had much less risk of heart problems, cancer, and diabetes; and lived years longer.

In 1990, medical science turned another page. That was the year when Dr. Dean Ornish showed that a plant-based diet, along with other healthful lifestyle changes, could actually reverse heart disease, causing narrowed coronary arteries to reopen without surgery. Meat-based diets—even "lean" meats—had none of that power.

At the Physicians Committee for Responsible Medicine, our research team put a plant-based diet to the test for diabetes, weight problems, and other health conditions. We found that when people threw out the animal products—meat, dairy products, and eggs—and powered their bodies with vegetables, fruits, whole grains, and beans, their health rebounded. Cholesterol levels fell, unwanted pounds melted away, blood pressure came back down, and diabetes came under much better control, sometimes disappearing altogether.

And the benefits go beyond human health. Environmental scientists have weighed in, showing that a plant-based diet does a huge favor for the Earth. Needless to say, the animals benefit, too. At the moment, Americans eat one million animals every hour. The more we chip away at that figure, the better off everyone will be.

So all in all, breaking the meat habit is just about the healthiest, smartest, and kindest thing you can do. If you are uncertain where to begin, this book will help you change your menu for the better. It will motivate you to begin the transition and will guide you along the way. I would encourage you to read it carefully, then share it with your friends. It will change their lives.

Neal D. Barnard, MD, President, Physicians Committee for Responsible Medicine Washington, D.C.

Introduction: Serving a Side of Truth

Food is part of the emotional fabric of American life. We celebrate at restaurants and socialize with friends over lunch. However, what we are eating for breakfast, lunch, and dinner represents today's global health and environmental crises. *The Meaty Truth* is here to serve us a side of the truth.

Our health has turned to sh!t as America is rapidly becoming the home of the sick and obese! About half of the illnesses claiming American lives are all related to what we eat. The USDA knowingly allows toxins such as arsenic, bleach, pus, and feces into our meat and dairy products. The crap fed to children in schools is a national tragedy. We are reaching the end of the antibiotic era and the rise of pandemic diseases is around the corner. Filthy, disease-breeding factory farms that churn out twenty-seven billion animals per year rely on consumer ignorance to keep pumping out meat and dairy products that are poisoning us and our environment.

Our heavily meat and dairy diets are decimating our entire ecosystem. Half the Amazon is expected to be gone forever by 2030. Dead zones are expanding so rapidly that they are predicted to entirely wipe out fisheries by 2048. Imagine oceans without fish. This is where we are heading. Our vital resources are running so low that experts predict the next world wars will be over access to water and food resources.

Fortunately, a healthy food movement is sweeping across America. The food system of our future is predominately whole grain, plant-powered food. While we were raised to believe that milk and meat are essential and vital components to a healthy diet, studies from around the world, including prestigious universities Harvard and Cornell, show that meat and dairy in no way constitute any part of a healthy diet. The truth is meat and dairy products are the primary cause for our alarming rise in chronic health problems and disease.

We understand that for some of you this seems crazy. Think about this: until 1863, slavery and the separation of people of different colors was an accepted practice in society. The ability to buy a human being based on race was not questioned and even supported by our government. In the early 1900s, women were to be seen and not heard. Doctors considered women too fragile to handle everyday pressures, and women were secondary members of society without a voice. In the 1940s and 50s, smoking cigarettes was recommended by doctors as an acceptable way to relax, open our lungs, and improve overall health. Smoking was sophisticated, even portrayed as sexy, and above all was just something everyone did, unquestionably. Over time, however, we challenged our assumptions and realized that these socially entrenched practices we believed to be okay were unhealthy and, in some cases, deplorable. We think drinking pus, eating animal sh!t, and fighting over clean water is simply unacceptable. This is happening in America every day. The time for change is now.

Right now we are heading down a path of destruction and disease. But, dear reader, you are taking the first step toward a happier, healthier, and more vibrant life by reading this book. We will set the record straight and let the truth be told. By the end of this book you will understand that *what is at the end of your fork is more powerful than anything in a pill bottle and more effective at preserving the environment than an energy-saving lightbulb or Prius.*

CHAPTER 1

The Disaster on Our Plates

Old MacDonald's farm, featuring happy cows and chickens on green pastures, is a fantasy of the past. In the 1960s, our meat and dairy production completely and quietly changed without the public's knowledge.[1] Familiar names such as Murphy Brown, Hebrew National, Knott's Berry Farm, Healthy Choice, and Good Nature Pork that line our grocery store shelves are all controlled by a small number of meat and dairy tycoons, such as Smithfield, Tyson, or Cargill.[2] This monopoly-like style control of the market by large corporations have pushed small family farms out of business. However, today's intensive and mass assembly-line production of meat and dairy products that focuses on quantity over quality is actually contributing to the debilitating rise in chronic diseases that are killing us and completely decimating our environment.

The Good Old Days Illusion

The twenty-seven billion animals in the United States that wind up on our plates are crowded into about twenty thousand warehouses or factory farms that dot the American landscape. (Governmental organizations commonly refer to factory farms as CAFOS, or concentrated animal feeding operations.) Ninety percent of the meat and dairy in our country comes from factory farms.[3] Just a handful of CAFOs are responsible for almost all of the meat we eat—95 percent of our chickens, turkeys, and pork and 75 percent of our beef products.[4] That's a lot of responsibility and trust placed into the hands of a few giant corporations. While these tycoons masquerade as family-friendly farmers, the reality is so far from the truth. Their concern for profits comes at a severe cost to humanity and America's health.

Most Americans have absolutely no clue where our food comes from and how it is produced. Factory farms thwart every attempt by the public to learn the facts about what exactly takes place behind the doors of their animal warehouses. Today, ignorance is so passé. It's high time we know the stinking facts about our food.

Let's trace how our food is treated before it is served on our plates. Today, value is placed on raising as many animals as possible in the smallest amount of space and within the shortest time span so they can be slaughtered at a laser-fast pace. The animals we eat are forced to live in crowded warehouses. Billions of animals exist in stalls too small for them to turn around or move and are forced to breathe in the stench of their own feces and urine morning, noon, and night. Twenty-four hour ventilation fans circulate the stench of all the other animals' crap. The ammonia levels are so strong that the chemical is traceable in the animal tissue that we eat. Contrary to what we see plastered on advertising posters of happy cows, these animals live out their short lives on cement floors without ever seeing the sun or grassy pastures. These inexplicably horrific conditions cause the animals' health to suffer, as well as ours when we eat those animals. Remember, we are what we eat.

In reality, factory farms are akin to poorly run hospitals. Imagine a hospital that is packed with patients who are lined up tightly side by side. The patients stand or lie in their own waste and urine. There is no staff to clean up. The patients are fed an unnatural diet that keeps them fat and sick. Everyone in the hospital is given antibiotics, whether they need them or not. Bacteria-resistant disease, many of which are antibiotic-resistant, then spreads easily from one patient to the next. The stench is unbearable, but there is no room to turn around or move. Every patient is stuck in filthy rooms with no escape. Doesn't look like a hospital we'd want to check into, does it?

This is what happens in factory farms to the twenty-seven billion animals raised for food each year. The filthy, primitive conditions are so severe the animals are continuously given therapeutic doses of antibiotics, anxiety pills, and painkillers to survive long enough for slaughter. Still thousands of animals go to their deaths with cancerous tumors and open, pus-filled sores, which are processed into the meat we eat.

The Perfect Storm: Setting the Stage for Disaster

How did the American farm become an industrial-horror machine? Technological innovation, unprecedented consolidation, the desire for "cheap" food, and the explosion of fast food restaurants created the perfect-storm opportunity for this disaster to take place. While hailed at the time as "progressive," cheap and unhealthy food produced in these disastrous conditions rather turned out to be a giant leap backward.

Meat and dairy food production is dominated by a few large companies—namely Smithfield, Cargill, JBS, and Tyson. The reality is the food we eat, more likely than not, is produced by one of these companies. Simply put, food is power. These large corporations figured out that if they could control all aspects of food production, they could control and generate more profit for themselves and their shareholders.

Moving from the Chicago Stockyards to the rural countryside where the local communities have no power to oppose them, corporations have contracted with local farmers to create factory farms. We may optimistically think that these corporations are creating jobs based on the contracts with these farmers. Wrong. They put these farmers into debt. The farmers enter into agreements enticed by profits and benefits they almost never see. The corporations' employees are required to front the costs for the factory farms, which are not cheap. The $700,000 up-front cost isn't pocket change for most farmers.[5] At the mercy of their binding contracts, these employees become controlled by the corporations from rising debt that keeps them in the factory-farming business. Since the market is heavily consolidated, it leaves little room for competition. The monetary value of the animals is completely in the hands of the corporations, which are able to manipulate the market to set prices. These farmers have only about one or two slaughterhouses to take their animals to and those costs are almost always set by the corporations.[6] We all know from basic Economics 101 that the ability to manipulate market prices is not capitalism and erodes fair competition.

Remember American History class where we learned about the Steel Trust, Sugar Trust, and Tobacco Trust monopolies in the early 1900s?[7] A few individuals controlled more than 55 percent of the markets in these commodities, limiting competition and wreaking havoc on the American ideal of capitalism. When the top four companies in any sector control between 40 and 45 percent of the market, these markets are considered consolidated. The Sherman Antitrust Act of 1890 was designed to bust these trusts and monopolies to allow for fair competition in the marketplace.

Today's agribusiness corporate structures sound all too similar to these historical monopolies. For example, in 1970 when farms were beginning to become factories, four meatpacking firms controlled only 21 percent of the beef market.[8] A 2009 Congressional report showed that the top four beef-processing companies controlled 71.6 percent of the market.[9] The poultry, dairy, and pig markets showed similar concentrations, each above 60 percent. The most recent study from the University of Missouri-Columbia in 2012 evidences that these sectors are only becoming more consolidated. The top four beef-processing companies now control 85 percent of the market.[10] Overall, the top four food and agricultural companies control 83 percent of the market. This is far from equal and fair competition.

The meat and dairy industries of today are dancing to the same tune as the earlier trusts and monopolies by dangerously limiting fair competition in the marketplace. Instead of the government the Sherman Antitrust Act to regulate the industry like the other trusts in the past, agribusiness lobbying efforts on Capitol Hill have made it possible for the livestock agriculture industry to effectively evade these charges. The hands-off approach the United States Department of Justice and the USDA have taken toward this unfair competition is shocking as it goes against the very core principles of fair markets that Americans pride their country on maintaining. Clearly, we need to look again at the definitions of "fair" and "capitalism" to reform our current food market.

Finally, the Obama Administration in 2010 proposed new antitrust rules that could add some regulation and teeth to the Stockyard and Packers Act. The goal of the Grain Inspection, Packers, and Stockyards Administration (GIPSA) "is to level the playing field between packers, live poultry dealers, and swine contractors, and the nation's poultry growers and livestock producers."[11] Well, it's about damn time. This actual attempt at regulation did not sit well with the meat, dairy, poultry, and pork associations. Mark Dopp, the policy director for the American Meat Institute, claims that "this rule attempts on many levels to undercut all the progress that's been made in the meat industry."[12] Representatives of Tyson and Pilgrim's Pride Chicken add that they view these rules as "one-sided" and "unrealistic."[13] Unfortunately, agribusiness can wield substantial legislative influence. The final rules issued in February of 2012 had lost most of its teeth in addressing anticompetitive practices.[14] We cannot afford to let these corporations continue to evade antitrust laws and erode the core of American business practices.

Dominating food production gives these companies unfair power economically, politically, and socially. Agribusiness corporations infiltrate the very organizations designed to regulate them and generously support government elected officials. Seems a little fishy, doesn't it? The agribusiness corporations even figured out a way to influence legislation, to limit what the public can access about what is actually happening down on the "farm." In fact, thirteen states have veggie libel laws that make it *illegal* to speak out against factory farming.[15] What happened to freedom of speech? Even Oprah Winfrey got sued because she merely stated that she would never eat a hamburger again after hearing how the animals were treated and what they were fed.[16] The fact that a corporation has the power to sue for expressing a personal opinion is troublesome. Corporations rely on keeping what happens on the factory farms out of the public's eye to maintain their business style. Unchecked and almost too big to fail, these corporations are allowed to set rules that harm animals, ruin our health, and destroy the environment. The problem is that the corporations are already failing us.

Technology: Friend or Foe?

Technological innovation does not always equal a better world. Bombs and warfare might be considered technological progress, but that doesn't mean they create a peaceful world. In fact, we view them as threats rather than as peacemakers. Similarly, factory farms might seem like progress, but they are in fact a threat to our health, finite resources, and the welfare of billions of animals. The innovations that made it possible to move animals from their natural outdoor homes to closed-in, filthy, and primitive conditions are not creating a better or healthier world. If anything, they have backfired. Factory farms are creating more problems by changing a once solar-powered, open-air farm into a carbon-powered factory: a perfect environment to breed pandemic viruses capable of wiping out whole populations, destroying our waterways, and using up our precious resources at alarming rates.

The purpose of factory farming is to produce the most animals in the least amount of space and time. By using massive quantities of soil-depleting fertilizer for feed crops, switching animals to an unnatural diet of grains, and overusing a slate of antibiotics, agribusiness corporations made it possible for factory farms to exist.[17] A farm animal's natural diet is grass from the outdoors. In a factory farm, they eat fattening grains. While grains are healthy for humans, soybeans and corn make animals severely sick because they cannot properly digest them. Instead of addressing this problem by giving animals their natural diets, the corporations are wasting research money on genetically modifying the stomachs and intestinal tracks of cows to have them digest grains. Crazy? We agree.

Today, most of the grain grown, about 80 percent, goes to feed animals raised for food rather than to feed humans. To keep up with the demand for grain, farmers overuse fertilizer that depletes and destroys the land and causes soil erosion while running off into our waterways. This means we need more land to grow crops. To produce more grain for the animals, about fifty-five acres of rainforest are destroyed each year for each pound of meat.[18] We can no longer sustain this level of catastrophic environmental destruction to feed the animals we eat. We are speeding toward disaster by continuing down this reckless path.

Remember swine flu? These superbugs are launching from factory farms since their tight quarters are the perfect breeding grounds for disease. To combat the dozens of potential diseases and bacteria in the area, the animals are dosed with a cocktail of the same antibiotics used to treat human illnesses.[19] This therapeutic use of antibiotics has created massive, antibiotic-resistant pandemics. We are even finding antibiotics in our waterways and in our fish.

Doctors, researchers, and international organizations warn that this ridiculous practice is making us rapidly approach the end of the antibiotic era.[20] While the FDA recognizes this looming threat, it has done little, if anything, to combat this problem. In addition, the FDA allows corporations to continue receiving genetically modified feed, growth hormones, and a long list of additives, including the same components used in warfare materials, fireworks, and bleach, that are not proven safe for public consumption. Why do corporations engage in these public health threats? Growth hormones allow animals to reach market weight in weeks rather than months. These growth hormones are notorious for triggering the growth of cancer cells. Feeding junk food and drugs to the animals is not helping us. Is this really technological progress?

Fast Food Factory

It isn't news that fast food burgers are not remotely healthy for us. All fast food meat, chicken, and pork come from animal factories. The infamous golden arches, along with Carl's Junior, Burger King, and other joints are one of the main reasons factory farming has managed to reach such high levels of corporate consolidation.

Factory farming and fast food go hand in hand; both are based on the same principle of serving massive quantities of really cheap food. It is no surprise that a large push to produce more animals to get into Happy Meals to feed our children as cheaply and quickly as possible came from this industry. This trend continues, as McDonald's is one of the largest purchasers of beef in the United States.[21] In the United States alone, McDonald's purchases 800 million pounds of beef and 725 million pounds of chicken per year, making its buying power huge.[22] It is also one of the largest purchasers of dairy, as McDonald's buys about 231 million pounds of cheese in a year. In total, this nine billion-dollar grocery bill is more than the entire United States' military food budget.[23]

Fast food companies desire to buy uniform cuts of meat to achieve the exact same-looking burger and chicken nugget sizes, all at very low prices. In the past, the processors would buy a few animals of different shapes and sizes from hundreds of regional farmers and small, family-owned farms. Cattle were openly bid on, allowing a competitive market.[24] But this system isn't ideal for ninety-nine-cent "finger-lickin'" chicken. These same-taste, same-size patties provided the incentive for meat processors to buy from only large and intensive producers to meet the fast food companies' demands. The quality of food, the cost of our health, and the condition of animals' lives is an entirely different story.

Behind Factory Doors: An Industrial Horror

Each year an estimated nine billion broiler chickens, 113 million pigs, thirty-three million cows, and 250 million turkeys are raised for consumption.[25] That is thirty million animals killed *per day*. Now is the time to pull open the factory doors and really see how our food is "raised."

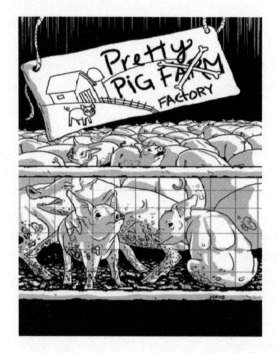

Let's start with how America's most popular meat—chicken—is produced. Walk into a shed in the Delmarva Peninsula where Kentucky Fried Chicken comes from, and you will see a 490 feet x 45 feet shed housing about thirty thousand broiler chickens. Imagine living in a space smaller than the size of an 8½-inch x 11-inch piece of paper. This is how much room each chicken gets for its entire life. There is barely room to breathe, and the animals are covered in feces and waste from other birds. The air is so thick with ammonia from urine that if it were not for the twenty-four-hour-required ventilation fans, the birds could drop dead on the spot from the level of poisonous gases. The level of toxic fumes is literally blinding. Ammonia is stored in the chickens' muscle tissues, which we will eventually eat.

In egg-laying operations, about six to eight chickens are crammed into cages that are stacked one on top of the other. To maximize space, the open wire cages, which are too small for the birds to move around in or spread their wings, are stacked on top of each other. For about two years, the chickens lay egg after egg until they are spent. They are so covered in feces and waste from the birds above them that it is hard to see a trace of their feathers. Chicken sh!t can pile as high as six feet in a warehouse, and inhaling the stench can feel as if your lungs are burning.

We have engineered chickens to become obese so quickly that they are not able to move; often their legs break because they cannot carry their own weight. It takes just forty-five days to grow a five-pound chicken, which is half the normal growth time.[26] Fatty grains and arsenic are the main ingredients to make the chickens gain weight at an unprecedented rate.[27] That's right: arsenic, a known poison, is in our food products. Just as added weight causes health problems for us, these birds also suffer from major health issues such as heart attacks and immobility. When these birds are taken to slaughter, most of them are deathly ill. *Ninety-nine percent of the chicken we eat comes from factory farms!* We are eating obese, toxic, antibiotic-ridden chickens, and it is no wonder we are getting sick. Still want those scrambled eggs for breakfast?

Pigs, the prized "other white meat," are subjected to a similar fate to become our Christmas hams and pork loins. The pigs are pumped with the drug ractopamine, which is banned in most countries, including China.[28] China is notorious for lax regulations, especially when it comes to animals, and even it doesn't accept this practice.

Pigs are crammed by the tens of thousands into close-quarter sheds, where they are forced to lie down in their own sh!t on cold cement floors, unable to even turn their bodies in another direction. Sows are confined in 7 feet x 2 feet crates, and their snouts are often covered in blood from being cut on the cage bars. These pigs' tails are cruelly amputated without any anesthetic. Pigs use their tails to communicate. This is the equivalent of humans having their tongues cut out. It is widely proven that pigs have the same level of intelligence as a toddler, and yet we can all agree that it would be considered severely abusive if we subjected our toddlers to any of this treatment. We wouldn't treat our family dogs and cats like this, even though science shows that pigs are smarter than dogs. We love our pets, so why are pigs any different? Our values are at odds with how we are treating these animals.

Thousands of cows are crammed together in feedlots where, instead of green pastures to graze on, they stand knee deep in their own sh!t, covered in flies.[29] Since there are usually about three people to oversee thousands of animals, open and festering sores on the cows' hides are left untreated. The truth is they are ground up and turned into our food. Appetizing, isn't it? There are hundreds of documented videos and articles that show downed animals, or animals too sick to walk, that are taken to slaughter and served up on your plate. We are making meat and dairy products from sick animals' carcasses, loading the meat products with dangerous toxins, and wondering why we are experiencing an unprecedented volume of epidemic health problems. It isn't hard to see that factory farming's horrific conditions are contributing to our rapidly declining health. It's really common sense.

Oh Baby, Baby, Baby!

Factory farm animals are baby-making machines. Ladies, imagine pushing one baby out, then getting pregnant again and again until your bodies collapse. It is a ridiculous practice. The sheer unnecessary volume of milk products produced each year come from cows that are subjected to a life of pregnancy to fulfill our milk and dairy desires.

Milk, the touted pure superfood, does not arrive on our shelves by magic. Instead of being milked by a farmer like in the good ol' days, dairy cows stand row upon row in their own waste, as machines hooked up to their teats consistently suck them dry.[30] But a cow's milk is *not* made for humans. It is a specific formula for a baby cow to grow about four hundred pounds in a short few months.[31] Sadly, the baby calves do not even get their mothers' milk. Instead, the female calves are given a formula, and the males are given a specific mixture stripped of iron to keep them severely anemic for that prized, white veal. Every mammal produces its own milk specifically to help its own babies grow. Despite advertising claims by the dairy industry, our bodies do not need and are not made to drink cow's milk.

On top of it all, dairy cows are given growth hormones to produce more milk, which often gives them an infection called mastitis. Mastitis produces pus that lands in our dairy products.[32, 33]Let's be clear here: we drink the pus. The shocking truth is the USDA regulations allow pus into our food products. This is not only extremely gross but unhealthy. Once the mothers' bodies give out from overuse, they are shipped off to slaughter, where they are made into our low-grade hamburger meat. The next time you sit down to dinner, think about what you are eating and where your food came from before it reached your plate.

Shutting the Factory Down

Corporations argue that factory farms are efficient, humane, and necessary for keeping the cost of meat down. They even call them progressive. But it is hard to call a place where blatant abuses, such as stomping on piglets, ripping off pigs' ears, cutting chickens' beaks, and kicking and hammering down cows is progressive or humane by any means. *Barbaric* is a better word. What corporations like to call efficient and cheap has come at a huge cost to our own health, the lives of the animals, and our environment as we turn our health, land, and water into piles of crap. While companies argue that reforming factory farms would be undoing progress, these factories have already taken us backwards economically, socially, and environmentally.

Know your Sh!t Solutions:

1) *Avoid the crappy factory-farmed food, especially fast food. Anything advertised as cheap, fast, and convenient food is equivalent to unhealthy. Seriously, it's filled with sh!t.*
2) *Find out where your food comes from, and don't be fooled by "home-grown" labels. "Cage-free" and "all-natural" meat are meaningless labels.*
3) *Start implementing Meatless Mondays.*

CHAPTER 2

America the Beautiful: From Cesspool to Shining Cesspool

Factory farming is turning America into a land of crap. It produces 1.3 billion tons of animal crap each year.[1] That is eighty-seven thousand pounds of manure produced *per second*.[2] This is the equivalent of 130 times the amount of crap per person in the United States, or five tons per person.[3] We have a colossal manure-management problem that is very inefficient and downright destructive. We know manure is by no means a sexy topic, but we have to address factory farms' overflowing cesspools that are creating mountains of manure that devastate our health and environment across the nation every day.

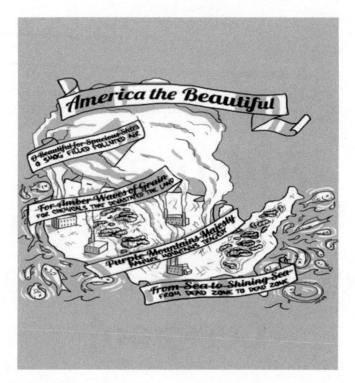

Imagine if all of our bathroom activities were flushed into our backyard pools for storage and just left there to evaporate. This is obviously disgusting to even think about and, at minimum, extremely unsanitary. But this is what is happening all across America on animal-factory farms. We are turning our beautiful homeland into a fetid swamp as thousands of cesspools the size of football fields, filled to the brim with animal manure, now cover the American landscape.

While hard to believe, this animal crap is the primary culprit in decimating our waterways: by wiping out our streams and our oceans, producing dangerous, toxic organisms that are killing off our fish, and causing major manure spills that make oil spills pale in comparison. Rivers once blue are turning brown and even unnatural colors, such as orange, yellow, and red. Our waterways are running red with blood from the billions of dead fish lining the banks of the rivers with open, oozing, bloody lesions caused by the virus *Pfiesteria*, which comes from animal crap dumped into our water.

Why is manure degrading our waterways such a problem? Well, the United States is already in a water crisis, and spilling crap into freshwater streams is only making matters worse. Major water wars are being fought from north to south and east to west for access to water. At a minimum, we should regulate to keep remaining water bodies as clean as possible. Yet there is little to no regulation from the Environmental Protection Agency (EPA), and agribusiness is getting away with dumping crap into our most precious resource. Ask yourself: what happens when all of our clean water turns to sh!t?

A Sh!tty Situation

Altogether, if the amount of animal crap from factory farms were packed into boxcars, there would be enough cars filled with manure to go around the whole world fourteen times![4] In terms of weight, that's over one billion tons of animal crap.[5] This is some heavy sh!t! This is more than *five* times the amount of waste produced by all of the people in the United States. Just one Smithfield pig farm in Utah that houses five hundred thousand pigs produces more sh!t than the 1.5 million people crowding the streets in Manhattan. The questions are where is all of this crap going and how damaging is it to our environment and our health?

Welcome to Cesspool Paradise

As the number of independent family farms has decreased in size, the number of animals per factory farm has substantially increased and so has the amount of manure in concentrated areas. For example, in 1975, there were more than 660,000 pig farms that produced about sixty-nine million pigs every year. By 2004, 90 percent of those farms had disappeared, but the number of pigs produced had risen to 103 million per year.[6] Today, the EPA estimates that there are about twenty thousand large-scale factory farms in the United States.[7] This means massive volumes of manure on a few farms.

The meat and dairy industries overlooked one very important detail when making the decision to house thousands of animals in one place— where do they put all of the mounds of untreated animal crap? Outside, pools of animal crap now line our beautiful countryside. The animal manure is stored in thirty feet deep, football field-sized holes in the ground. One factory farm can have hundreds of these so-called "waste disposals." The corporations call these holes in the ground *lagoons*, giving off the image of a tropical paradise. This is quite a misnomer. The animal manure is so toxic and densely concentrated in these holes that the crap turns from brown to a salami-pink color.

Let's be honest. Sticking liquid manure into holes in the ground seems like a primitive form of getting rid of waste. This is the type of sanitation, or lack thereof, that organizations work to remedy in countries without first-class infrastructures. The underlying rationale for this disposal method is to allow the manure to sit there and evaporate. No, we aren't making this up.

One of the many problems with this "logic" is that manure contains ammonia, which is a toxic type of nitrogen that is released as a gas when the manure is left to decompose in the open-air lagoons. About 70 to 80 percent of the nitrogen in the liquid lagoons changes into ammonia. As a gas, ammonia can travel more than three hundred miles through the air before it is dumped back onto the ground and into water sources. Let's put this into perspective: it takes about five to six hours to drive three hundred miles. That means ammonia emissions in New York can be in Massachusetts in half that time. Since ammonia is the most potent form of nitrogen, it triggers eutrophication, which causes harmful algae blooms that wipe out marine habitats.[8]

This gas is just the beginning of our problems. Manure contains 160 noxious gases, including deadly hydrogen sulfide.[9] As air pollution, and especially ammonia, can travel for hundreds of miles, this is no longer a local problem; anyone can be affected. Health concerns associated with ammonia include chemical burns to the respiratory tract and chronic lung disease. Just two minutes of exposure to ammonia "may result in chronic lung disease, and massive exposure to ammonia can be fatal."[10] Air pollution was apparently not a high concern when deciding upon this disposal method.

Imagine a major city of more than twenty thousand people without sewage-treatment plants. It seems ironic that we would spend so much money on sanitation methods for human waste and yet nothing on animal waste when there is three times as much coming from these factories. In contrast to human sewage, which is carefully treated and highly regulated, manure from factory farms is not. Think about this: there are 160 volatile organic compounds emitted in liquid pig crap. Unlike industrial waste and pollutants, for some peculiar reason the vast quantities of animal manure is not regulated. This means the animal waste remains in its highly toxic form.[11] The biological oxygen demand, or BOD, of liquid manure is 160 times that of raw, municipal sewage. So not only is the manure not treated, but it is also more toxic. Logically, this does not make sense.

Not to mention, animal manure is densely polluted with lethal toxins, blood, heavy metals, bacteria, and oxygen-depleting nutrients, such as nitrogen and phosphorus from animal feed, hormone injections, and antibiotics that are given to the animals.[12] This turns into a deadly combination for us and our environment.

Did you know we can get more than forty different (and many deadly) diseases from animal manure? These anaerobic lagoons that dot our landscape are terrible at eliminating any sort of pathogens, heavy metals, or the BOD that severely affects our waterways.[13] Fifteen percent of viruses and 55 percent of bacteria survive in the lagoons and easily leak into water sources.[14] Foodborne illnesses currently affect about one-third of our population. These foodborne pathogens are up to one hundred times more concentrated in animal manure than in human waste.[15] For the very reason that just *one* gram of hog sh!t can carry up to one hundred million fecal coliform bacteria, where and how manure is stored directly impacts our personal health, biodiversity, and the health of the environment. We can't put off dealing with this stinkin' problem any longer.

Sh!t Sprinkler Systems

Back in the days of small, family farms, we applied manure to the land to fertilize it. This natural recycling process is impossible now because there is simply so much sh!t we cannot put it all on the land. Now we house the crap in man-made slurry lagoons. Each one of these lagoons holds about twenty to forty-five million gallons of liquid, animal manure.[16] But the volume of manure even exceeds these massive holding capacities. In fact, a study by the University of Northern Iowa found that "if farm workers had applied manure at the rate at which the crops could have absorbed phosphorus, the CAFOs would need more than nine times the field area used for manure application by these CAFOs."[17] The problem is that manure contains too much nitrogen and phosphorus for the land to absorb.

Overapplying manure to the land turns not only our farmland but also our waterways into crap, as manure runoff contaminates nearby rivers and streams, creating dead zones that kill marine life. An EPA investigation in Yakima Valley found "brown streams of manure running directly into ditches and creeks."[18] Kendall Thu, a noted researcher, found that at any CAFO where there is more wastewater than the surrounding land can absorb, water contamination from overapplication is almost guaranteed.[19] Mr. Thu found that there was a direct relationship between water-quality problems and the dairy operations in the area. Water pollution from overapplication is exacerbated during the winter. When the land is frozen, it cannot absorb any manure, which all becomes runoff. This runoff causes severe problems. For example, in 2009, twenty-five thousand gallons of manure that were overapplied on a farm field in Mitchell County, Iowa, produced runoff that killed 150,000 fish in a four-mile stretch of a local stream.[20]

Overapplication and the resulting water contamination is a common practice with poultry production. For example, in 2009, the Waterkeeper Alliance sued a Perdue farm in Eastern Shore, Maryland that allowed an uncovered pile of chicken manure to drain into a tributary of the Potomac River. The manure not only increased the nitrogen levels, but also the *E. coli* and fecal-coliform levels—bacteria that cause human-health problems and may be fatal.[21] The Delmarva Peninsula is home to the highest production of boiler chickens and eggs in the nation. The over application and runoff of manure is considered one of the main contributors to the growing dead zones in the Chesapeake Bay and the degradation of its waters.[22] The Chesapeake Bay is an American landmark and vital waterway. It is time to stop factory farms from sh!tting in it!

Amazingly, between football field-sized cesspools and over-application of crap to the land, there is still a problem of keeping the crap levels in lagoons down. So what do the corporations do? They came up with a brilliant idea. When the lagoons are full and the land is similar to a swamp, factory farmers will illegally spray the manure straight into the air, without a care as to where the manure falls. That's right: they created sh!t sprinklers.

Local families have come back to find their homes covered in the sticky, brownish mist of crap and their trees dripping with feces. Helen Reddout, a cherry farmer in Yakima Valley, surrounded by eighty-five mega-dairy farms, provided a devastating image of how our land is going from green to brown and even black. She states that "when you go to bed at night the grass is green. When you wake up there is just black slime everywhere." There is zero retribution for the destruction of property. Families in California have had to fill in and remove their swimming pools because they too frequently turned into mini cesspools. The stench is so severe that it permeates everything—from clothes and bed sheets to car interiors. People drive to work dry heaving, with eyes watering from the stench of sh!t. As one farmer proudly stated, this reeking odor is "the smell of money."[23]

On the other US coast, in North Carolina, the Tar Heel State, the Waterkeeper Alliance sampled and measured water near pig farms and found that the muddy-colored water was in fact animal crap that had been sprayed into the air. This is happening across America.

Aside from the blatant destruction of property, shooting manure into the air is a public-health hazard. One woman surrounded by dairy factories in Yakima Valley walked out of her house one morning and inhaled sharply due to the horrible stench. The ammonia in the air permanently burned her vocal chords, and her voice is now just a rasp. The Yakima Valley also boasts some of the highest rates of asthma and cancer compared to the other counties in the state. We doubt this is just mere coincidence. In fact, four comparative studies of asthma in children living near and farther away from factory farms clearly indicate that those children living near factory farms have higher asthma rates.[24]

Repeated exposure to the particulate matter in manure can cause chronic bronchitis, decreased lung function, and even heart attacks. However, the EPA doesn't seem interested in the obvious health concerns associated with factory farming. Although factory farms are supposed to be regulated under the Comprehensive Environmental Response, Compensation, and Liability Act (CERCLA, also known as the Superfund Act), the EPA decided to exempt factory farms from reporting their emissions. Instead the EPA instituted a voluntary Air Quality Compliance Agreement where factory farms monitor their own emissions. The catch is that the EPA doesn't suspend or sue offenders, but merely slaps on a small fine that doesn't even dent the corporations' pocketbooks. This whole process seems a little backwards.[25]

Needless to say, these current "solutions" are crappy. It is just plain wrong to allow these corporations to pollute our air, land, water, and private property without any retribution or accountability for turning America into a land of deadly, smelly cesspools.

Leaky Lagoons

Factory farms' cesspool paradise is seeping into just about everyone's backyard. On top of manure being illegally sprayed and over applied on the land, lagoons are notorious for leaking, spilling, and flowing into every stream, river, and groundwater source. Families across the country are turning on their taps to find brown, disgusting, foul liquid pouring out instead of the clear water they were anticipating from their private wells.

While the corporations will advise that the lagoons are perfectly safe and have a lining to prevent seepage, their statements remain completely unsupported. Many of the cesspools are not lined, but even if they were, lining becomes weak as it deteriorates over time. The average life span of a lagoon is only about twenty years, if kept in optimal shape.[26] The majority of the lagoons, however, are around much longer, because, again, there is the problem of where to put all the crap if the lagoons are no longer used.

While seepages and leaks can be reduced by using clay liners in the lagoons, studies have found that even clay-lined lagoons can leak anywhere from "several hundred to several thousand gallons per acre per day."[27] Lagoons with lining can seep about one million gallons of manure. One reason is due to decomposition. The gases produced from decomposing manure cause the liners in the lagoons to swell, which forces tons of feces out of the lagoons and into our land and waterways. Liners are not foolproof. Polyethylene liners, which are commonly used to house pig crap, are easily punctured by rocks in the ground, providing an open door for the animal manure to seep into your groundwater.

A famous, Pulitzer Prize-winning, in-depth 2006 study, "Boss Hog," found that nearly half of all lagoons leaked enough to pollute wells, aquifers, and nearby springs.[28] "Boss Hog" first called attention to the issue of leaking lagoons in its exposé of North Carolina's industrial swine production. One corporation, Carroll Farms in North Carolina, tested nearby wells next to three of its factory farms. It found that the ammonia levels were "ten times more than the normal level of two parts per million" and continued to increase over time, but Carroll Farms dismissed this obvious level of toxicity.[29] Carroll Farms's dismissive behavior is not the exception but the norm. Corporation after corporation today continues to throw their hands in the air and fail to act on the blatant evidence of their lagoons poisoning the surrounding environment and putting the lives of thousands of Americans at risk.

We have to hand it to agribusiness for the superb placement of these lagoons right above aquifers or in flood plains surrounding local, family homes. Over four and a half million families in the United States are at risk of nitrate pollution because they get their drinking water from groundwater, whose purity is threatened by leaking lagoons. When nitrogen breaks down in manure it forms nitrate, which can leach into groundwater and drinking water.[30] Nitrate pollution is a serious public-health risk.

Since "today, over one million people are estimated to take their drinking water from groundwater that shows moderate or severe contamination with nitrogen-containing pollutants, mostly due to the heavy use of agricultural fertilizers and high rates of application of animal waste," the continuous, nutrient pollution from animal crap poses a serious public-health risk.[31] When nitrate gets into drinking water, traditional forms of cleaning the water do not work. It requires a special treatment that costs about $4.6 billion and comes out of your tax dollars.

In 2005, the Illinois River watershed, which provides drinking water for twenty-two public-water systems in Oklahoma, contained a phosphorus load from poultry productions nearby equivalent to the waste from 10.7 million people. This level is more than the entire populations' of Oklahoma, Arkansas, and Kansas combined.[32] In California, officials have identified agriculture, specifically the dairy operations, as the main source of nitrate pollution in more than one hundred thousand square miles of polluted groundwater for drinking.[33]

More than making the water taste bad, 2012 studies confirmed that nitrate contamination in our drinking water is associated with increased risk and incidence of thyroid cancer.[34] Nitrate exposure in drinking water nearly doubled the risk of cancer in men. However, even disinfecting the water produces a catch-22 situation. The disinfectants that get the nitrate out of our water have been consistently linked to an increased risk of bladder cancer.[35] Think about this: about forty-five million Americans get their drinking water from private wells.[36] More likely than not, the majority of this population is located in rural areas more susceptible to factory-farm contamination.

Nitrate contamination is known for causing blue baby syndrome, among other health problems.[37] When Gordon Kelly, the head of the Yakima Valley County Health Department, was informed of the high nitrate levels and manure water coming out of private wells in the California area, his response was, 'well, the nitrates just affect infants.' Reassured by Mr. Kelly, we can all sleep soundly knowing that just the health of our babies and next generation is in jeopardy from these consistently leaky lagoons.

Manure and Oil Spills

In 2010, the BP oil spill in the Gulf of Mexico made the front pages of newspapers for weeks, as images of the disaster took over the nightly news. The CEO of BP was put under tremendous scrutiny for the accident that sent 4.9 million gallons of oil into the Gulf. There was a public outcry, and hundreds of groups helped to clean up the spill. The BP oil spill was larger than the infamous 1989 Exxon Valdez spill, which impacted 1,300 miles of ocean and killed an astounding 250,000 birds. Why are we talking about oil spills?

While oil spills receive nationwide coverage and public outcry, consistent lagoon spills occur all the time with zero nationwide and limited, if any, local coverage. Some of the lagoon spills are comparable to, if not bigger than, the Exxon Valdez spill. For instance, in 1995 a 120,000 square-foot lagoon at Oceanview Farms in North Carolina burst, sending twenty-five million gallons of feces and wastewater into the New River.[38] The spill killed at least ten million fish and polluted 350,000 coastal acres of shellfish habitat. Dead fish began lining the banks of the river within two hours of the spill. The manure sludge was so dense it took two months for the sludge to make the sixteen-mile stretch down the New River to the ocean.

While the Oceanview Farms spill is *double* the size of the Exxon Valdez oil spill and considered the largest environmental spill, we are pretty sure most Americans have never heard of it. Neither, at the time, did citizens who were swimming in the river downstream. The government officials failed to warn them of the hog crap contaminated with *E. coli* heading their way. We highly doubt the same protocol would have been followed if it had been an oil spill. The Oceanview Farms spill has gone down in history as one of the greatest environmental disasters, which killed every living creature in its path in the North Carolina waterways.[39] The Oceanview spill was bad enough, but that same year, three lagoons in North Carolina burst within two weeks of each other.[40] One smaller lagoon spill occurred on the same day as the Oceanview spill in Sampson County. The other spill in Duplin County released nine million gallons of chicken waste into Limestone Creek, which is a tributary of the Northeast

Cape Fear River.[41] In comparison to oil spills, which rarely happen at the level of the BP and Exxon Valdez spills, lagoon spills are consistent, frequent, and pose comparable environmental damage with less coverage and support.

According to the National Resources Defense Council, "from 1995 to 1998, one thousand spills or pollution incidents occurred at livestock feedlots in ten states and two hundred manure-related fish kills resulted in the death of thirteen million fish."[42] Not much has changed since that time.

In 2001, an Illinois contract farmer refused to lower his lagoon by at least a million gallons of manure. Instead, the owner, Dave Inskeep, decided to fill a nearby ravine that was dammed with a ten-foot berm with two million gallons of the manure. The lagoon didn't hold and sent millions of gallons of feces rushing into the Kickapoo Creek, which joins the Illinois River. It was one of the worst avoidable spills in Illinois history.[43] Fast forward to today, and we can see that for some reason we are not taking lessons from the past when it comes to manure spills. For example, did anyone hear about two three-hundred-thousand-gallon manure spills in Wisconsin in 2013? One of these massive spills, while an "accident," produced a mile-long trail of animal waste.[44] Why did this accident happen? There weren't proper berms in the holding tank and pipes. Apparently it just wasn't cost effective to install them, even though manure spills create devastating and sometimes-irreversible environmental damage. What is even more frustrating is that the corporation responsible for this mess only received a slap on the wrist and a thank you for alerting the Department of Natural Resources (DNR) to the problem, despite the fact that this spill was illegal.

If only the cycle of spilled crap would end. But the trouble is manure spills are becoming ever more frequent. In fact, there were a total of seventy-six manure spills in 2013 alone in Wisconsin, totaling more than one million gallons of manure.[45] This is a 65 percent increase in manure spills from 2012. In an attempt to provide some assurance, Kevin Erb, the manure specialist at the University of Wisconsin-Extension, proudly claimed that the volume of manure spilled "is minute compared to the amount of manure cows produce. The spill total for 2013 is less than 1 percent of all the waste produced by dairy cattle in Wisconsin."[46] This news somehow isn't as consoling to us as Mr. Erb probably hoped.

Worse is the industry's attitude to the manure spills. According to Tom Bauman, the Coordinator of Agriculture Runoff at the DNR, "Spills are going to happen."[47] We don't agree with this laissez-faire attitude when CAFOs do not have to exist at all. Spills have lasting consequences. After a manure spill in Pennsylvania in 2013, the city had to close down a children's playground indefinitely because *salmonella* and other pathogens were simply not decreasing.[48] Since we would never allow children to play in a playground of crap, why are we okay with eating it in our food?

Fortunately, a coalition in Iowa, sick of constant manure spills, decided to take a stand and sue The Maschhoffs, one of the largest pork-owning networks in the country. The coalition filed the suit for violating the Clean Water Act after the fifth manure spill since 2007. Already Iowa has 630 polluted waterways from manure and climbing.[49] While The Maschhoffs claims innocence and states it is a "good neighbor," its multiplicity of spills speaks otherwise. Its Keosauqua Sow Unit has dumped more than twenty thousand gallons of manure into the Des Moines River and surrounding tributaries.[50]

The Maschhoffs has provided the typical-industry response by stating that this claim filed in November 2013 is without merit. And yet as Lori Nelson, the Iowa Citizens for Community Improvement Action Fund board president, stated, "Every factory farm in Iowa is a ticking time bomb that could have a spill at any time, and the DNR needs to start holding them accountable for polluting our waterways by issuing them Clean Water Act permits so they have to follow stronger environmental standards." Why are we not regulating "ticking time bombs"?[51] Instead of accepting the fate of manure spills, is it such a novel idea to prevent them or even find real solutions?

Swimming in the Slurry

It might seem laughable that we are concentrating on animal crap, but the truth is that this overload of sh!t is causing us some stinking problems. The Environmental Protection Agency (EPA) states that factory farming has so severely damaged over 170,000 miles of rivers and streams, 2,500 miles of lakes, and 2,900 miles of estuaries that they are no longer safe for hosting recreational activities or sustaining the surrounding wildlife.[52] In California alone, the National Resources Defense Council found that animal crap is responsible for polluting more than one hundred thousand square miles with nitrates and pathogens. Untreated manure waste from factory farms is responsible for polluting thirty-five thousand miles of rivers in twenty-two states and additionally contaminating our groundwater supply in seventeen states, according to the EPA.[53] The scary part is these numbers do not reflect all the waterways in the United States. The extent of the damage is unknown. Maybe it is time we begin crying over spilled manure.

The primary pollutants of concern for water quality are nitrogen and phosphorus, the most abundant nutrients in animal manure. The United Nations (UN) study, "Livestock's Long Shadow," indicates that livestock is the largest contributor to increased nitrogen and phosphorus levels.

Whoever thought that tons of nutrients could be bad? Nitrogen and phosphorus are actually essential nutrients to life. But the abundant quantities that manure produces prove deadly. The impacts of excessive nitrogen and phosphorus nutrients are enormous, from "drinking water contamination, toxic and non-toxic algae blooms that impair recreational waters and kill fish, changes to coastal-marine fisheries, acidification of soils and terrestrial and aquatic ecosystems, and increases in ozone and particulate matter that can harm human health and damaged productivity of crops and forests."[54] Nutrient pollution is such a serious threat to our streams, lakes, and rivers that "farms have now replaced factories as the biggest polluters of America's waterways."[55]

Nitrogen and phosphorus from manure are forever changing our landscape as they kill off our waterways and all the life in them. Let's look at what happens when too much nitrogen and phosphorus get into our waterways from manure. Excess nitrogen and phosphorus deplete the biological oxygen demand, or BOD, in the water, which causes more plants and algae to grow.[56] This is called eutrophication. When eutrophication happens, desirable fish species are replaced by less desirable species and algae, which feed on the oxygen, causing economic costs to fisherman, shifts and drastic changes in aquatic habitats, production of toxins that cause harmful algae, clogged irrigation canals, and death—both for aquatic habitats and fish.[57] The Pagan River in North Carolina, which runs by a Smithfield Foods hog facility, provides a chilling picture of the water damage from manure and nutrient pollution. The "Pagan had no living marsh grass, a tiny and toxic population of fish and shellfish and a half foot of noxious black mud coating its bed. The hulls of boats winched up out of the river bore inch-thick coats of greasy muck."[58] This is in addition to the river turning shocking colors of red, orange, and pink from the high contamination levels.

Aside from the grim picture, the most significant consequences from nutrient pollution are the creation of dead zones and the ignition of the presence of a deadly "cell from hell" that also poses human-health risks.

The "Cell from Hell"

During the massive lagoon leaks and spills in North Carolina in the mid to late 1990s that sent millions of tons of manure into the rivers, residents were noticing fish belly-up in the rivers with strange marks on them—open sores that were oozing with pus. Fishermen who spent their lives in the water and came into contact with the river water began to develop the same pus-filled sores that wouldn't go away. No matter what antibiotics were used, the sores stayed open. Then these fishermen began to experience memory loss, forgetting simple things like how to get home; some even had trouble breathing. No one could explain these mysterious human-health effects or what was killing the fish.

Dr. JoAnn Buckholder, a researcher at North Carolina University, uncovered the silent killer named *Pfisteria piscicida*. *Pfisteria* is an odorless, invisible, silent, fish-killing dinoflagellate, which, like any good assassin, only leaves its trail of dead as the mark of its presence. In this case, *Pfisteria's* mark is a trail of dead fish. *Pfiesteria* "degrades a fish's skin, laying bare tissue and blood cells; it then eats its way into the fish's body—leaving open sores as the main tell-tale factor."[59]

Dr. Buckholder found that *Pfisteria's* presence is directly linked to manure's presence in the water from nutrient contamination. Nutrient overload causes the perfect conditions for toxic algae growth or *Pfisteria*. This "cell from hell" has been seen at factory-farm hot spots such as the Chesapeake Bay and particularly in North Carolina after massive lagoon spills. *Pfisteria* left nearly twenty million fish dying with open sores from this massive disaster.

While the species of *Pfisteria* still continue to stir up debate among scientists, one thing is very clear: *Pfisteria* is a killer that has been shown to eat human blood cells. Humans exposed to *Pfisteria* develop the same bloody lesions on their skin that fish do, but also experience neurological problems such as memory loss as well as "severe respiratory difficulty, headaches, blurry vision, and logical impairment."[60] Other problems include immunological and musculoskeletal conditions as well as an acute burning sensation on the skin.[61] When manure starts producing a "cell from hell," one that can potentially mutate into a deadly monster, it is a strong indication that something needs to change.

Graveyards in the Oceans

Imagine an ocean without life in it. This is where we are heading, and fast. The pollutants and contamination from manure spills and dumping into our waterways is killing whole aquatic ecosystems by creating dead zones, areas where life cannot be sustained. As we mentioned earlier, eutrophication contributes to and is a leading cause of dead zones, which are typified by the decay of algae that depletes oxygen levels. This may lead to hypoxia (low oxygen) conditions that make it impossible for living creatures to survive, as they cannot support the oxygen demand for aquatic life.[62]

Dead zones are currently lining the coasts of America's once-pristine shores. Dead zones are a direct example of the impairment of waterways by nutrient overloads that are a result of agricultural wastewater runoff. The most notorious 22,126-square-kilometer dead zone in the Gulf of Mexico, equivalent in size to the state of New Jersey, is the dumping ground for the Mississippi River, which passes through the heart of agribusiness in the Midwest.[63] While the Mississippi River is historically a dumping ground for industrial waste as well, the Council on Environmental

Quality of the White House Office of Science and Technology Policy found that animal manure alone contributes 15 percent of the nitrogen to the Gulf of Mexico, while industrial and municipal waste only contribute about 11 percent.[64]

The number of dead zones in the United States has increased from twelve in 1960 to three hundred today. According to a 2010 White House Report, this rapid devastation of our marine life "poses both economic and environmental hazards."[65] The increasing number of skeletal remains of once-abundant and unique aquatic life is a precursor to the further destruction of our marine life if positive steps are not immediately implemented from agribusiness.

This Water Tastes like Sh!t

The quintessential summer days of jumping into the river out back or drinking the water from your own well are long gone. Manure is so pervasive that we can catch *salmonella* poisoning from swimming in a river or merely ingesting some of the water! Manure carries pathogens and antibiotics that threaten our health as they contribute to antibiotic resistance and the spread of waterborne diseases. The presence of fecal-coliform bacteria in the water indicates the presence of *E. coli* and manure in the water.

Research by the USDA Agricultural Research Service reveals that *E. coli* is not only alive and well, but also living in a streambed near you. How comforting. Agricultural runoff causes *E. coli* to leech into surface water, as well as set up a home in streambed sediments. Since *E. coli* can live for months and years in these sediments, longer than it can on surface water, it poses a latent human-health risk of waterborne diseases when these sediments are disturbed.[66] This means swimming in your local stream during the summer could land you or your kids in the hospital with *E. coli* poisoning. For the record, *E. coli* and *salmonella* are polite euphemisms for crap. These pathogens strike fast and hard; they kill thousands of people every year and permanently disable thousand of others, shutting down and liquefying vital organs.

What Happened to the Clean Water Act?

It would seem that with the growing concern and increasing number of troubled waters that the EPA would act. The Clean Water Act is the primary piece of legislation that monitors factory farms.[67] It was passed by Congress in 1972 with the intent to "restore and maintain the chemical, physical, and biological integrity of the nation's waters." Under this act, CAFOs are designated as point-source pollutants, meaning they are operations that discharge pollutants "directly into waters of the United States."[68] Yet the industry has failed time and again to enforce the Clean Water Act. Up until 2003, it was not a federal requirement that factory farms obtain permits to pollute the waterways. The EPA and Department of Agriculture only issued regulatory guidelines for the first time in 1998 due to the public outcry from the infamous North Carolina lagoon spill.[69]

Currently, most CAFOs remain unregulated, and even if they are regulated, discharge permits serve little to no purpose. Under the EPA's rules, if a factory farm plans to discharge crap into nearby streams, it has to have a permit. Let's be clear: factory farms are *allowed* to pollute as long as they have a piece of paper that says they can. This is probably why the EPA has failed to curb pollution. In addition, the EPA does not set hard-and-fast rules for how much CAFOs can discharge.[70] This voluntary "polluters' permit" strategy does very little to mediate current pollution or deal with the underlying problem—the massive amounts of manure.[71] When it comes to corporations adhering to environmental standards, a voluntary approach is just not going to cut it.

The EPA's Office of Water reported that approximately nineteen thousand CAFOs require permits, but only 8,300, or 43 percent, have discharge permits.[72] Given these numbers, there are about eleven thousand factory farms that are discharging waste unregulated. Clearly, this system is completely unsustainable. Fortunately, the EPA recognized its lack of progress and declared factory farms a "national priority." However, the EPA is still stuck focusing on compliance for discharge permits, not on providing actual penalties that would force compliance. Compounding this problem, the Clean Water Act only provides a federal foundation for establishing rules; it is up to the states to enforce them. As each state has varying rules, our nation's current approach to remedying our water and environmental crisis from factory farms has proven haphazard and ineffective. Friends, the giant corporations keep raking in money while we, the taxpayers, are left footing the bill for cleaning our water sources. More importantly, we are running out of time to act.

All hope is not lost. Favorably, there have been instances where citizens have been able to push through state regulations that better protect our water sources and curb agribusiness's extensive political clout. Consider New Mexico: Jerry Nivens, a concerned citizen who could no longer stand to see his waterways polluted, organized a petition that ended in New Mexico passing some of the most progressive dairy-water regulations to date. The dairy industry is the largest agricultural sector in New Mexico and has a strong influence in Congress. Yet, it also is responsible for polluting 60 percent of the state's groundwater, where 90 percent of the people in the area get their water.[73] Although the dairy industry put up a four-year fight against the regulations, Nivens and his team forever changed New Mexico law—showcasing that everyday citizens do make a difference.

Get Ready for Water Wars

Leading international organizations predict that the wars of the future will not be over oil, but clean water. Already there are hundreds of legal suits in the United States over rights to freshwater use. These water wars are just the beginning, because visibly clean water is a foundational necessity for all living beings to survive. Currently aquifers are being drawn at extreme rates—250 times their ability to refill. Already the twelve-million-year-old Ogallala Aquifer is predicted to run dry within in the next twenty years from overuse and abuse by the livestock industry.[74] With only 1 percent of freshwater available and a growing population of over seven billion, our water resources are strained at best, without having manure destroy what we have left.

As excessive amounts of liquid animal manure can easily access our waterways and drinking water, we stand to bankrupt not only our health but also one of the Earth's most valuable and cherished resources—*clean water*. Waterways are a core component of the life cycle, and without our aquatic habitats, our whole ecosystem is doomed to fail. The frequency with which manure is contaminating our water sources and poisoning our groundwater that millions of us use for drinking water is now a nation-wide problem. We need to deliver immediate and swift remediation and force agribusiness once and for all to clean up their sh!t.

Know your Sh!t Solutions:

1) Animal crap is now in everyone's kitchens and backyards. Clean your fruits and veggies.

2) Filter your water. Beware of swimming in rivers, lakes, and streams.

3) Speak out against factory farms in your area! Each voice counts. Don't want to be living next to a cesspool? Sign a petition! Raising our voices in unity can make these corporations liable for their messes.

CHAPTER 3

Seriously? You're Still Sick?

"The doctor of the future will no longer treat the human frame with drugs, but rather will cure and prevent disease with nutrition."

~ Thomas Edison

It is well known that America's health has drastically turned to sh!t. We like to pride ourselves on a fantastic health-care system with state-of-the-art research facilities and renowned doctors. While all of this may be true, the fact remains that we rank as one of the sickest countries among the industrialized nations of the world. As a nation, we are on the cusp of an evolutionary health disaster. Something has got to change.

Today, 70 percent of deaths in this country are attributed to chronic diseases.[1] These diseases were almost unheard of a mere one hundred years ago. The leading chronic conditions such as heart disease, cancer, arthritis, Alzheimer's, and diabetes used to be confined to an aging population, as evidenced by their definition as "degenerative" chronic diseases. Yet now we are seeing them in an increasing number of school-age children.

This generation of children has the highest rate of health problems, including obesity, diabetes, attention deficit disorders, and autism. One in three children are obese, and this is the first generation of children who will have shorter life spans than their parents. Today, one in two Americans die from heart disease, one in eight women are diagnosed with breast cancer, and the chance of being diabetic in America is now one in three.[2] Although we turn to technology to "fix" our health problems, we are no further ahead in our quest for wellness.

So where are we going wrong? It is really quite simple. We are heavily consuming the wrong foods. In the 1900s, Americans got 70 percent of their protein from plant-based foods. Today we get 70 percent of our protein from animal-based foods.[3] Americans consume more meat per person than anywhere else in the world.

As meat and dairy prices have fallen, we have moved to gorging on animal products and processed foods while fruits, vegetables, and whole grains have been largely relegated to the sidelines. We have essentially switched a diet filled with fiber and nutrients and low in cholesterol to one high in saturated and trans fats and cholesterol and devoid of fiber. It is not surprising then that as our meat consumption has nearly doubled and our dairy consumption (particularly of cheese) has quadrupled since the 1950s, so too have our waistlines, health problems, and health-care costs. We have twice the obesity rate, twice the rate of diabetes, and three times the cancer rate than the rest of the world.[4] Although we love to blame our genetics or look to the "history of disease" in our families, it's time we look at our All-American recipes.

We Aren't Meat-Eaters!

Most people can agree that factory-farmed meat is bad for our health. (If you don't, we suggest you reread Chapters One and Four.) Laden with genetically modified organisms, toxins, chemical fillers, growth hormones, ractopamine, arsenic, and antibiotics, this meat is a recipe for health problems. This growing knowledge has spurred nationwide campaigns for "local," "grass-fed," and "organic" beef. While these are nice sentiments, the problem is that meat by its very nature is a disaster for our health. The added toxins are just the icing on the cake. The reality is that we were never meant to subsist on meat.

We are led to believe that eating meat and dairy are the building blocks for good health. We think we are doing right for our bodies by filling up on lots of animal protein and drinking cow's milk. The Paleo Diet is the newest fad that professes we are designed to be meat-eaters. Really? Where did they get that idea? Although the Paleo Diet does rightly state that we need to eat more natural and less processed foods, the fact is that meat is actually not natural for humans to consume.

Our bodies are designed to live on plant-based foods. We are actively poisoning ourselves every time we eat animal products, whether they are 100 percent local and grass-fed or from Smithfield's industrialized factory.

Why are meat and dairy so bad for us? In short, meat and dairy are pro-inflammatory—meaning they produce inflammation. Inflammation is the genesis of every chronic disease. Just like we strive to keep a balance between work and play, our bodies need to maintain an optimal pH balance (slightly alkaline) to be healthy. Meat and dairy are highly acidic and disrupt this balance, creating an ideal environment for disease to thrive. Cancer loves the acidic environment created by a meat and dairy diet. Every bite of meat and dairy is akin to a drop of poison that our bloodstreams carry throughout our bodies—affecting each and every system, from our respiratory, immune, and endocrine to our musculoskeletal. Additives from factory farms such as growth hormones and antibiotics are just added abuse.

Let's examine some important anatomical differences between us and carnivores that place us firmly in the herbivore category. If we compare carnivores, omnivores, and herbivores, our anatomy most closely resembles that of plant-eating apes and chimpanzees. Firstly, we have blunt teeth, not fangs for ripping meat. Most carnivores are capable of swallowing ripped chunks of raw meat whole. If we tried to do the same, we would end up choking. Secondly, we have long digestive tracts, whereas carnivores have very short digestive tracts.[5] When we eat meat, it putrefies in our digestive systems, leading to disease. With a short digestive tract, natural carnivores avoid meat putrefying in their colon and digestive tract.

Finally, we aren't meant to function on protein, especially animal protein. Despite marketing myths, protein is not the most efficient or effective energy source. In fact, protein often tires us. Many of us have experienced a "food coma" after a heavily animal-protein meal. What are our bodies most efficiently designed to process? Carbohydrates. That's right. Unlike carnivores, our stomachs produce amylase, an acid used to break down carbohydrates found in plants. Marketing has pitted carbohydrates as the enemy, but the truth is that our bodies thrive on glucose from carbs. This is the energy that fuels our brains. This does not mean we can eat cake all day. The type of carbohydrate is important. We need complex carbohydrates like whole grains for energy.

For over fifteen years, it has been well established in medical literature that just one meal high in animal fat, such as a typical American breakfast of sausage, scrambled eggs, and cheese, can damage our arteries.[6] When our arteries become inflamed, they are less flexible and become stiff. It takes about four to six hours for our body to combat this inflammation. By that time, it is already time for lunch. When we continue to eat meat and dairy products, we flood our body with acid, creating an acid overload. It is a vicious cycle that keeps our bodies in a perpetual state of chronic, low-grade inflammation that sets the stage for disease, one meal at a time.

Today, doctors, not just in the United States but from around the world, are confirming that our compounding health-care problems and escalating health-care costs are primarily linked to our consumption of meat and dairy products. Study after study and physician after physician (who aren't paid by the meat and dairy corporations) are showing that dairy and meat products are *disease-producing*. Four out of the ten leading causes of illness and death in the United States are linked to our meat and dairy-based diets. A mere three-ounce steak can increase our risk of dying by 13 percent![7] Researchers at both Harvard and Cornell University issued statements saying that the optimal amount of meat in our diets is *zero*!

Our high rates of chronic conditions stem from our decision to directly go against our plant-eating roots. We can think of our bodies as cars. We can fill our tanks with soda, and the car will run for a while, but eventually it will malfunction. Similarly, we can feed our bodies the wrong fuel, but eventually they will break down.

Let's review three of the most common American afflictions: heart disease, cancer, and type 2 diabetes, to see why we can ditch the pills for plants.

The American Diet Is a Heartbreaker

Too many of us think that heart disease is our fate. Popping cholesterol pills has become the new normal. In the United States alone, six hundred thousand people die each year from heart disease, and there are five hundred thousand new cases each year.[8] The American Heart Association estimates that heart disease will cost the United States $818 billion dollars in health care per year by 2030.[9] Our health-care system might not be able to keep up with this astronomical climb in disease. Consider this: almost all males over fifty-three and females over sixty-six who have grown up eating the traditional American diet are already suffering from some form of heart disease.[10] An even bigger problem is doctors are now seeing hardening of the arteries, a disease called atherosclerosis that is a precursor to heart disease, in children as young as eleven.[11] Most of us don't even realize we have heart disease until we suffer a heart attack or stroke. More worrying is that most first heart attacks are often fatal. The real tragedy is that heart disease is completely preventable. This "household" name should not even exist.

Heart disease is really a misnomer, as the entire body, not just the heart, is affected. Know this: if you have clogged arteries anywhere, you probably have clogged arteries everywhere. For example, guys, having a problem getting it up? One of the first signs of heart disease in men is erectile dysfunction. As we travel south, our arteries get smaller, making the penal arteries the first to be affected. Although companies have created billion-dollar empires around this "soft" issue, pills are only temporary solutions to your sexual woes and won't help your heart either. Want to fix your bedroom problems? Take a hard look at your "manly" meat-and-dairy diet.

In simplest terms, the cause of heart disease is plaque or fatty deposit buildup in the sixty thousand miles of veins and arteries throughout our body. Healthy arteries are lined with a smooth substance called endothelial tissue and are supposed to be strong and elastic. When we eat foods high in fat and cholesterol (i.e, meat, dairy, eggs, cheese, and butter), these endothelial cells become sticky and fatty deposits, or plaque, stick to our arteries and accumulate. This buildup of plaque is like the narrowing of a hose pipe. Eventually it slows blood flow and causes hypertension. A heart attack happens when this plaque buildup eventually ruptures and spills toxic contents into our bloodstream. In response, our platelets try to come to the rescue and fix the problem, but their help can actually deprive our heart muscles of vital oxygen, resulting in a heart attack or, in some cases, sudden death.

Let's be crystal clear on the issue of cholesterol: excess cholesterol that forms plaque *only* comes from animal products. Plant-based foods do not have cholesterol. Researchers around the world have proof that eliminating animal protein from our diet can reverse and prevent heart disease. One landmark study—the Framingham Heart Study—demonstrated that lower cholesterol levels can protect a person from cardiovascular disease.[12] Similarly, the renowned Dr. Caldwell B. Esselstyn Jr.'s twelve-year study was one of the first to show the protective qualities of a plant-based diet.[13] Of his eighteen subjects who followed this diet, none of them had cardiac events over the twelve years. Those that did not follow the diet continued to have cardiac events over the same time period. Not one drug, diet, or surgery has been able to replicate the same track record.

Thousands of Americans undergo risky bypass surgery, have stents placed, or live on cholesterol medication. For whatever illogical reason, simple solutions like dietary changes are considered more radical than having our chests cracked open. The bigger problem is that surgery and pills do not address the underlying cause of the disease. Think of your heart like a tire with a hole in it. We wouldn't keep pumping air into the tire and driving on it in the hopes that it would magically fix itself. We know the tire would inevitably blow out, so logically we would change the tire. In this case, we can't put a Band-Aid on heart disease with medicine; we have to fix the underlying cause, which is where the plaque is coming from in the first place.

For those skeptics out there that think we can't "solve" heart disease through diet, let's look at what would happen if we actually cut back on animal protein. Fortunately, one country decided to try this experiment. In the 1970s, Finland's mortality rate from heart disease was the highest in the world. (Sound familiar to America's current heart disease epidemic?) In an effort to reduce heart disease, Finland's government decided to cut back on all animal products, including meat, eggs, and dairy products. To gain support, the government implemented nationwide programs that reduced intake of saturated fat from cheese, chicken, cakes, and pork. They even assisted in switching dairy farmers to berry farmers. The result? There was an 80 percent drop in heart-disease deaths, and cardiovascular and cancer mortality was cut in half.[14] This drastic change was from just reducing animal-product intake, not completely eliminating it. Impressive? We think so too. Heart disease doesn't run in our families but rather in our family recipes. The mounting evidence is clear. We have the answer. It's our choice between pills or plants. We will opt for the plants, please.

The Dirty "C" Word

An increasing number of families are devastated by cancer, especially hormone-related cancers such as breast and prostate cancer, each year. In the United States alone, there are 146,000 new breast cancer cases and forty-six thousand deaths from breast cancer each year.[15] In the past this was something that only happened to postmenopausal women. Today it is now afflicting women in their early twenties and thirties.

Put simply, cancer is a faulty replication of our genes that mutates quickly if fertilized by carcinogens and unregulated. While genes do play a role in cancer development, what most people do not know is that diet can control our genes and essentially turn cancer on or off. All of us have cancer cells present in our bodies. Whether or not the cancer is expressed is determined, in many cases, by environmental and lifestyle factors such as diet. In fact, studies show that our genes play a very small part in our risk factor for cancer development. Only about 2 to 3 percent of all cancers are purely genetic. This means our chance of having cancer is primarily due to lifestyle and food choices. Cancer can be slow to manifest, meaning our childhood eating habits can set the stage for adult cancer.

Animal protein is one of cancer's best friends. Animal protein, such as that found in meat, dairy, and eggs "changes our hormone levels, modifies vital enzyme activities, causes inflammation and cell proliferation and creates an acidic atmosphere in the body—all of which create an ideal environment for cancer to thrive."[16] Friends, our current diet is cancer-causing. Simply put, the more animal products we eat, the higher the probability we have of getting cancer.

The World Cancer Research Fund recently reviewed over seven thousand studies and declared processed meats dangerous for human consumption, as they can cause cancer.[17] These include All-American favorites such as bacon, sausage, sandwich meats, and pepperoni. Why are these meats in particular cancer causing? Sodium nitrate used to give hot dogs that reddish color and MSG added to give a savory flavor to otherwise dead meat are known carcinogens or cancer promoters. Most Americas consume these foods every single day. Think one hot dog won't hurt you? Think again. Studies find that fifty grams of processed meat, the equivalent of one hot dog per day, increases the risk of colon cancer by 21 percent![18] We can cut our risk of cancer by as much as 40 percent by eliminating meat and animal products from our diet.[19] According to Harvard University studies, our risk of colon cancer drops by two-thirds if we stop eating meat and dairy products.[20] Who knew diet could be so powerful?

Studies are also finding that it is not just eating meat that is cancer-causing. Cooking it produces carcinogens as well. On every menu or USDA guideline, we are constantly reminded that undercooked meats could be harmful and cause foodborne illnesses. However, it's quite a catch-22, because cooking meat to the high temperatures required produces heterocyclic amines, or HCAs, which are known carcinogens. Cooking, grilling, frying, and oven broiling beef, pork, chicken, and fish even at normal temperatures produces these harmful mutagens. In particular, grilled chicken, which is touted as the "healthier white meat," has been found to contain some of the highest concentrations of HCAs.[21] Clearly, from cooking to eating meat, participating in this American habit is a significant cancer risk that we should rethink.

In particular, Dr. T. Colin Campbell has found that the most relevant chemical carcinogen identified is casein, the animal protein in cow's milk. Casein makes up 87 percent of dairy products. Every time we reach for a glass of milk, slice of cheese, or a cottage-cheese breakfast, we are instigating cancer growth. This is because dairy is not only acidic but also contains the natural growth hormones' insulin-like growth factor 1, or IGF-1, that stimulate growth and consequently cancer proliferation. For example, studies have found that when IGF-1 is dripped onto human breast cancer cells, the mutated cells grow uncontrollably.[22]

The silver lining is that removing meat and dairy from our diets protects us from cancer. The Pritikin Research Foundation studied the blood from participants on different types of diets and found that those who consumed a plant-based diet in comparison to the typical meat and dairy-based SAD (Standard American Diet) had blood that was less hospitable to cancer.[23] Blood from completely plant-based participants fought prostate cancer eight times better than those consuming meat and dairy products. Even better, in a mere two weeks a vegan diet was able to slow down and in some cases stop the progression of breast-cancer growth! Eating a plant-based diet can change about five hundred genes, "turning on genes that prevent disease and turning off genes that cause breast cancer, heart disease, prostate cancer, and other illnesses."[24] Ominously, the World Health Organization forecasted that the cancer rate will reach as high as twenty-two million cases a year over the next two decades.[25] Prevention rather than treatment is our best option to combat these numbers. It looks like we need to start eating a plant-based diet and run for the cure with banners promoting the power of plant nutrition.

Don't Blame the Sugar

Type 2 diabetes is becoming a national epidemic, especially among children. Since World War II, the rate of diabetes has increased by 700 percent, doubling almost every year for the past fifteen years since 1975.[26] The chance of a newborn baby becoming diabetic later in life is now one in every three. In the United States, diabetes alone cost $245 billion dollars in 2012, a 41 percent increase since 2007.[27]

Diabetes is a serious problem. It is the leading cause of blindness in the United States and is associated with an increased risk of heart disease. Other problems include nerve damage, cognitive decline, kidney failure, and amputations. The good news is that we can avoid losing our eyesight and save our kidneys by cutting the crap out of our diet.

Type 2 diabetes comprises 90 to 95 percent of diabetic cases in the United States.[28] Since type 2 diabetes is directly related to obesity, it means our current diabetic epidemic is lifestyle related. In fact, cross-cultural studies can depict a diabetes map of the world. Those places that more closely follow America's blind lead on diet have the highest rates of type 2 diabetes. America, we are self-inflicting this disease. This means we can stop it.

There has been a national outcry about the weight of the nation's citizens, especially as it relates to diabetes and childhood obesity. In school nurse's offices around the country, you can find insulin needles in every trash can as type 2 diabetes rates soar among children. Most of the efforts to address childhood obesity, such as the First Lady's "Let's Move" program, Katie Couric's movie *Fed Up*, and New York's move to ban supersized soda drinks, are well intentioned, but missing the larger picture. If anything, these efforts reiterate the lack of information surrounding the root of our health-care problems.

We think of diabetes as strictly a sugar problem. While diabetes is caused by elevated sugar levels in the bloodstream, the underlying cause is fat, hence its relationship to weight. In simplest terms, fat blocks our insulin receptors in the muscles, which pushes glucose into our blood-streams and leads to an excess of sugar.[29]

Most medical and dietary guidelines for diabetics strictly focus on limiting carbohydrates, fruits, and sweets. The problem is that they continue to allow people to eat excessive amounts of animal protein and foods high in fat, which only serves to promote, rather than control, diabetes. No offense to the American Diabetes Association (ADA), but its guidelines have yet to reverse diabetes in those who follow it nor does it incorporate the scientific knowledge we know today. Continuing to eat chicken and turkey high in cholesterol will not help regulate your blood-sugar levels. Diabetes does not have to be a life sentence. Yet most people are told that they have to spend the rest of their lives controlling or managing their diabetes. Seems like a lot of work to us. Luckily, there is a better way.

By reducing fat intake, we can unclog insulin receptors and allow insulin to function normally again. A landmark study in 2006 found that those eating a low-fat, plant-based diet were better able to control diabetes and, in many cases, reverse their diabetes than those following the ADA guidelines.[30]

No More White Lies

What about dairy? Isn't that natural at least? Every mammal has evolved to use the milk from its own mother to grow. Yet humans are the only species that chooses to drink the milk of another species. Nature never intended for us to continue drinking milk after weaning. This is why lactose intolerance is so pervasive around the world. After weaning, we naturally lose the enzyme that breaks down lactase in our bodies. Despite what we have been led to believe, cow's milk was not part of our ancestors' diet, and especially not in the amounts we consume today. We have been drinking milk only for the past six thousand years, which in evolutionary terms is the blink of an eye. Our bodies are not designed to consume cow's milk. According to Harvard University studies headed by researcher Walter Willet, "Humans have no nutritional requirement for animal milk, an evolutionarily recent addition to the diet."[31]

Of all foods, most people think that dairy is a perfect food for our health. Based on this assumption, Americans consume massive amounts of cheese, yogurt, milk, and other dairy products thinking that we are providing our bodies with a superfood. We have to hand it to the dairy companies when it comes to marketing. Dairy is a wonderful growth mechanism and the perfect food for baby cows. But dairy is the most imperfect food for human health, and it is linked to a host of health problems, including but not limited to: acne, arthritis, breast cancer, prostate cancer, ovarian cancer, heart disease, diabetes, autism, Crohn's disease, Parkinson's disease, and osteoporosis.[32]

That's right, dairy actually doesn't build strong bones. If dairy did promote strong bones, then the United States wouldn't have such high rates of osteoporosis and brittle bones as it currently does. We know this information goes against everything the dairy industry has been proclaiming for years, but "Got Milk?" doesn't translate to "Got Strong Bones?" In fact, our obsession with calcium from dairy products actually weakens our bones and damages our joints. A more apt advertisement for the best sources of calcium would be "Got Kale?" or "Got Broccoli?" as these foods are superior to dairy products. Dairy products rich in saturated fat, hormones, toxins, industrial pollutants, and both natural and artificial growth hormones might just be one of the most contaminated and toxic foods that we could eat. (For more on what's hiding behind dairy's angelic façade, read chapter six.)

A Weighty Problem

Eating healthy has become synonymous with lean-meat meals, the latest workout regimes, such as P90X and CrossFit, and calorie counting. Yet with every new fitness regime, diet pill, or diet fad such as Atkins, South Beach, or Weight Watchers, our waistlines have collectively continued to rise. Two in every three Americans are overweight and one in three Americans are obese. Just fifty years ago, only one in eight Americans were obese. If we were to look at the rise in obesity next to the rise in factory farms, the trends would mirror each other—an obvious relationship that our industries and government choose to overlook for the sake of promoting animal foods. Instead, marketing campaigns focus on sugary drinks and exercise. We use the gym as a place to "work off" our meals instead of keeping our bodies fit. Exercise is not the problem, collectively. Our increasing waistlines are directly linked to our heavy consumption of foods high in saturated fat and cholesterol, primarily from animal-based and processed foods.

Let's take grilled chicken, the most advertised lean meat for "healthy" eating, as an example. According to recent data in Europe from the EPIC study, one of the most comprehensive studies on nutrition, grilled chicken is not correlated with weight loss, but rather weight gain. Interestingly, but not surprisingly, the study found that weight loss was most associated with the decrease of meat consumption. Since obesity is the gateway to chronic disease, it is critical that we keep our weight in check. This is second nature on a plant-based diet, as it is low calorie and low fat. We can eat as much delicious food as we want and not have to count calories. Isn't this the ideal diet we have been waiting for all along?

The American Ideal is SAD

For some reason, society has correlated eating meat and dairy as a sign of wealth. American culture that prominently features the Standard American Diet of excessive meat and dairy meals is an ideal that most citizens of other countries desire to replicate. When populations that previously had lesser financial means come into money, the first thing they do is change their diets to mirror the American one. Flattering? Why yes. Healthy? Far from it. Within a generation, these populations get their wish: they mirror the American diet and the health problems that go along with it.

For example, in the 1950s, the Marshall Islands were awarded a substantial sum of money from the United States after it tested a nuclear device there. The citizens went on shopping sprees and completely changed their previously plant-based diets to meats, cheeses, and fish. Until the 1950s, diabetes had been relatively unheard of in the Marshall Islands. The Marshall Islands now have some of the highest diabetes rates in the world.

Our high rate of disease is a homegrown problem that stems directly from our fast-food, high-meat, and processed-food diet. Studies on immigrants from China and Japan, raised on diets mainly consisting of rice and vegetables, show that within a generation of moving to the United States and adopting our SAD diet, those immigrants experience the same rates of prostate cancer! It's hard to face these facts, but we can't deny the science.

If America is one of the sickest countries, then what does one of the healthiest countries look like? The Blue Zones Project sought to answer this question. Researchers looked at societies that had the highest longevity around the world and found that those who lived the longest, such as the Okinawans in Japan and the Seventh-Day Adventists in Loma Linda, California, largely ate an almost completely plant-based diet.[33] The question then is: is a plant-based diet really the healthiest or are there other cultural factors at play? Fortunately, there are rebels in every group, and the Seventh-Day Adventists have provided the ideal environment to actually test, as accurately as possible, how diet affects disease. The findings are astounding—those who stuck to the rule and avoided meat and dairy were the healthiest.[34] The rebels who ate more fish, eggs, meat, and dairy had higher rates of heart disease, cancer, and diabetes.

Ditch the Junk Science

Since the 1970s, the government has been attuned to the fact that eating animals is a disaster for our health. As we steadily became overweight and saw an increase in heart disease, President Nixon organized the Committee on Nutrition and Human Needs, led by Senator George McGovern, which researched three questions: Why are we getting sick? Why are we getting fatter? Why is heart disease increasing?[35] The committee's conclusion was that eating animals is bad for our health. So why has this information not been disseminated in society? Good question. When the committee came out with this recommendation, the meat and dairy industries had a field day and lobbied Congress. Along with voting McGovern out of office, the industry didn't just stop Congress from issuing a statement concluding that our meat and dairy diets were the culprits of our rising rates of disease; they also passed food libel laws that made it illegal to say certain foods are bad for our health. We aren't kidding. This happened. These food libel laws are still in effect today in one-fourth of the states.[36]

The meat and dairy industries have responded in full force to allegations against the harmful effects of their products. The animal-food industry even created the "Meat Myth Crushers" website to address the growing scientific literature that implicates animal foods as the primary culprits in our growing health crisis.[37] One of the main issues they push to sell their product and discredit health claims is that we need animal protein. Ounce for ounce, we can get more protein (without side effects) from roasted pumpkin seeds.

The industry claims that the site seeks to remedy the problem that most Americans get their information about food from the news, media, books, and movies. According to the meat and dairy industries, these somehow aren't credible sources. We are interested in learning how their site is apparently more credible and represents no conflict of interest.

The USDA's *Dietary Guidelines for Americans* is a prime example of industry sabotaging our health. Nine of the thirteen committee members issuing the most recent *Dietary Guidelines for Americans* all had ties to the food industry.[38] These guidelines are the foundation for the USDA's new MyPlate food "pyramid" that sets the federal nutritional standards and programs. Installing people on boards that have conflicts of interest is an American pastime for the animal-food industry. Current USDA Secretary Tom Vilsack has ties to Monsanto. Gregory Miller, the president of the Dairy Research Institute, also serves as the Committee Chair for the American Society for Nutrition.[39] Seems a little biased, doesn't it?

This is why meat and dairy continues to be featured prominently on the USDA food pyramids. However, these food pyramids, ingrained into us since grade school, were designed as marketing schemes straight from the Dairy and Meat Councils. In fact, the studies promoting meat and dairy are *paid for* by the corporations themselves. Statistically, the research funded by an industry is four times more likely to reach a conclusion supporting that financial backer. Knowing that fact, consider this: the dairy council spends $58 million a year on marketing and research.[40] That is a lot of studies showing the "benefits" of dairy.

Today other food pyramids designed by doctors put meat and dairy as the lowest priority on our plates or completely eliminate them. In fact, Harvard researchers do not endorse the USDA's guidelines at all. They call out these guidelines as fundamentally flawed and rather "intense lobbying efforts from a variety of food industries."[41] We tend to side with Harvard on this one.

The various meat and dairy councils and associations have a particularly close relationship with the very institutions we turn to for nutritional guidelines. Corporate sponsors of the Academy of Nutrition and Dietetics (formerly the American Dietetic Association) include the National Cattlemen's Beef Association and the National Dairy Council. As the nation's health spirals downward, one would expect leadership from the Academy of Nutrition and Dietetics, the world's largest organization of food and nutrition members, boasting over seventy thousand members. Yet this organization that should be promoting our health is completely infiltrated by the very industries it seeks to regulate. For example, at the 2012 Food and Nutrition Conference and Expo, about 23 percent of the speakers had undisclosed ties to food industries.[42] One of the most prominent sponsors is Coca-Cola, which oversees educational programming for the Academy. What was their take-home message? Teaching kids that sugar is not unhealthy and aspartame, a known carcinogen that also happens to be in some of their products, is perfectly safe. Clearly this is sound (and unbiased), nutritional advice for our nation's children.

For over a decade, the Academy has enjoyed continued financial support from food giants such as ConAgra Foods, General Mills, Nestle, and Kellogg's, as well as the National Cattlemen's Beef Association.[43] In particular, the Dairy Council is a premier partner and supporter. The "consume more dairy" message remains continuous year in and year out at the expo. Yet humans' zero necessity for dairy is completely at odds with this propaganda. The Academy is supposedly a prestigious organization that holds merit and weight on scientific publications about our food sources. As the Academy has been hijacked by corporate interests promoting unhealthy food at odds with science, so has its credibility.

It's not our fault that we have been eating wrong. It's also not our doctors' fault either. Doctors receive little to no education in medical school on the connection between diet and disease. Think about this: at one time, doctors endorsed smoking cigarettes. They recommended smoking to their patients to open their lungs and to improve overall health. Today this advice seems ridiculous. So why did the doctors promote it? First, there was a lack of information, and second, some doctors were paid by the tobacco corporations to promote their brand products.

The exact same phenomenon is happening with meat and dairy. Big pharma pays some doctors to keep their patients popping pills, and most doctors know very little about nutrition. Additionally, the USDA's mixed messages on what to consume leave consumers and, sadly, even our physicians wondering which message is right. For instance, the USDA website's "key message to consumers" is to switch to fat-free or low-fat milk.[44] Yet when milk is stripped of the fat, all that is left is sugar and the cancer-causing casein protein.

Clearly, this isn't healthy. More worrisome is that the USDA's website lists under health benefits of dairy possible prevention of osteoporosis and definite promotion of bone health. The site also claims that "intake of dairy products is also associated with a reduced risk of cardiovascular disease and type 2 diabetes, and with lower blood pressure in adults."[45] Really? These recommendations in no way match the plethora of scientific research that states the opposite. Fortunately, more and more doctors are waking up to the fallacy behind eating meat and dairy. Many now know that plant food, loaded with antioxidants and phytonutrients, is our best prescription for good health.

We are approaching an age where we have to take an active role in our health. According to the Centers for Disease Control and Prevention, fifteen of the sixteen leading causes of disease are lifestyle related.[46]

Friends, this is why our health-care system is broken. Our health is being bought by corporate interests. We can't afford to keep traveling down this path of misinformation and poor diets. For too long we have fallen prey to marketing schemes that confuse us and don't let us think for ourselves. We are smarter than this.

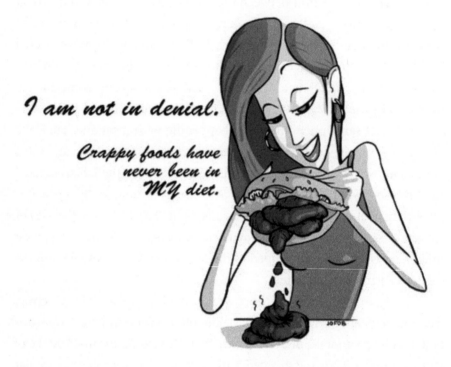

These largely preventable chronic diseases are consuming 75 percent of our national health-care budget.[47] Consuming animal foods generates over $600 billion in health-care costs every two years. Consider this: the notorious tobacco industry only generated $400 billion in health-care costs over the course of five decades.[48] We have admonished the tobacco industry and forced them to pay for their costs on our health. Why aren't we doing the same with the animal-food industry?

We are putting dead, rotting, obese (and more likely than not, sick) animals into our mouths. How is that going to help us? The reason we feel like crap is because we are eating it! We aren't supposed to live on prescriptions. Remember, what is on your plate is more powerful than anything at the bottom of a pill bottle. We have the answers to our health problems. It is time we make smart investments, and our bodies are our greatest investment. The power to change this paradigm rests on the end of our forks.

Know your Sh!t Solutions

1) *Stop eating crap and you will stop feeling like crap! Eliminate meat and dairy from your diet as much as possible. Keep in mind that our bodies cannot differentiate between free-range and factory-farmed meat. Even though factory farmed meat has added harmful toxins, any type of meat damages our bodies when you eat it. Go meatless every Monday and completely meat free by taking out meat from your diet one meal at a time.*

2) *Eat more fruits, veggies, grains, and legumes. Eating a plant-based diet does not mean living on salads. Shake up your meals and try new recipes.*

3) *Get Informed. Read* 21-Day Weight Loss Kickstart *by Dr. Neal Barnard,* The China Study *by Dr. Colin T. Campbell, and* Rethink Food: 100+ Doctors Can't Be Wrong *by yours truly! We have over one hundred doctors from around the world all finding the same answer—the key to a disease-free, healthy life is a whole-food, plant-based diet.*

CHAPTER 4

Scary Sh!t

"Just being honest, I don't think your average consumer probably knows a lot about how food is produced."

~ Elizabeth Hagen, USDA's Head of Food Safety

Pink slime made headlines in 2012 as we shockingly discovered that the majority of our hamburger meat was not only doused with ammonia nitrate—a common component in bombs, fertilizers, and detergents—but also was made up of ground-up, otherwise-inedible beef scraps and cow-connective tissue that could be highly contaminated with the lethal pathogens *E. coli* and *salmonella*.[1] This disgusting beef product referred to as "finely textured beef" comprised our children's school lunches and infiltrated our grocery stores. In fact, the US government was buying seven million pounds of it for school lunches.[2] As much as two-thirds of our ground beef contained pink slime and didn't require labeling. Even though food companies tried to pass off this chemical as non-toxic and benign for our health, let's cut the crap: even if ammonia doesn't kill us on the spot, we should not be eating it. Thankfully, public uproar forced three of the four lean, finely textured beef plants to close, as most major supermarket chains and school-lunch programs refused to buy their products.

The bigger problem is that ammonia is not the only toxin in our food. The stunning truth is that untested growth hormones, arsenic, a wide spectrum of antibiotics, anxiety pills, flame retardants, bleach, animal crap, chemical fillers, and pus are all *allowed* in our meat and dairy by the USDA and FDA. That's right. We eat *all* of those in our food products. Since this is not advertised or labeled, we have absolutely no idea what chemicals our food contains. These dangerous chemical fillers and toxins are catastrophic for our health. Imagine if every American knew what they were really eating how the industries would be forced to change their habits . . .

Spicing It Up!

Our food products are so loaded with chemicals and toxins that today we could liken them more to science experiments.

Ever wondered what autolyzed yeast extract is? It's monosodium glutamate, notoriously known as MSG. It is only one of the worst possible toxins that we could ingest. MSG is a known excitotoxin that stimulates our cells to the point of death. It is ubiquitously used in fast foods, and most of our processed food products. It is a known silent killer.

How did MSG get into our food supply? The FDA allowed it. This isn't to say this practice is remotely safe. The FDA Commissioner that promoted the benign health effects of MSG to Congress cited four studies. Turns out two of these studies didn't exist and the other two studies were incomplete.[3] And yet, the FDA still allows this known health hazard into our food supply. In fact, the FDA allows about three hundred foods to have secret ingredients—meaning the food companies are not required to specify them on the labels. It is high time we rethink how our food is produced.

Let's take a brief look at a small sample of some of the added "spices" in our foods.

- Penicillin: Yes, the same antibiotic given to us when we have strep throat is also in our food products. Antibiotic resistance, anyone?
- Arsenic: In ancient times, arsenic was used to poison one's enemy. Food for thought.
- Copper: Why do we need metal in our food? Recent studies show excess copper is associated with increased risk of Alzheimer's disease.[4]
- Sulfuric Acid: Also used to manufacture fertilizer and oil, sulfuric acid is found in lead-acid batteries.
- Sodium Hydroxide and Potassium Hydroxide: Both are prominent ingredients in soap and dishwashing detergent. There is a better way to eat "clean."
- Chlorine Gas: This sh!t just got real. This is used to make bombs in warfare. It is also widely used in cleaning supplies as a disinfectant.
- Hypobromous Acid: Who wants to drink bleach?
- Glyphosate: This is the most common herbicide used in Monsanto's Roundup. These toxins get in our food when animals eat their genetically modified feed. The result? It is known to damage our DNA and cause cancer in humans.[5]
- Sodium Nitrate: This is used in rocket propellant, smoke bombs, and fertilizers. Apparently preserving the bright-red color in processed meats like bacon and hot dogs is more important than not feeding us known carcinogens. Nitrates also affect how our body processes sugar, which can increase the risk of diabetes.
- Benzoate Preservatives: Although the FDA classifies this ubiquitous preservative found in many of our packaged-food products as "generally recognized as safe" (GRAS), sodium benzoate is also a main ingredient in fireworks.
- Natural and Artificial Flavorings:
  Who likes the taste of coal-tar derivatives? No, we aren't kidding. This is the best example of a science experiment gone wrong.

Flavorists can now make anything taste like it is grilled, smoked, or cherry flavored. The only difference between natural and artificial flavors is how they are extracted and created. The problem? This cheap mixture of chemicals that do not have to be spelled out on the labels can actually affect our RNA, which plays a vital role in gene expression.[6] We are introducing a concoction of cheap, man-made materials into our bodies and crossing our fingers for the best. Why is this allowed?

Please note that this is just a teeny, tiny sampling of what is allowed into our food products. The entire list of chemicals would completely fill the pages of this book.

Do you recognize any of these on our food labels? All of these chemicals and toxins do not have to be labeled. What's worse is that for many of these drugs, the USDA audit report found that the FDA has yet to set "tolerance" limits. For example, copper does not have a tolerance limit. The newest research implicates copper as one of the main metals related to the onset of Alzheimer's disease.[7] As we well know, Alzheimer's disease has no cure.

While the USDA and FDA claim these so-called ingredients are added in such finite amounts that they have no real effect, it seems our health problems are saying the opposite. There is absolutely no reason we should be eating bleach, disinfectant spray, chlorine, warfare materials, poison, and antibiotics. There is a reason most household cleaning products and detergents state to contact poison control if ingested. It seems ironic then that it is okay to consume these same chemicals in any amount during breakfast!

Drug and substance residues in your meat and dairy products can cause a range of reactions from skin lesions to nerve poisoning and death. We have never experienced such food-related health problems or food allergens before today. As most of these added chemicals are man-made, our bodies have zero experience or history processing these chemicals. Our food is now a disastrous experiment gone very, very wrong. A USDA audit report admits, "Since consumers have no easy way of protecting themselves against the residues of harmful substances in their food, it is

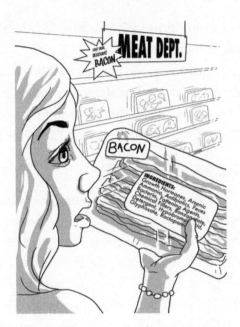

important that the national residue program's controls be as robust as possible to prevent meat contaminated with harmful substances from reaching the kitchen table."[8]

This could not be more of an understatement.

Is that Safe to Eat?

The American Farm Bureau Association proudly boasts, "Today's farmers produce 262 percent more food with 2 percent fewer inputs (labor, seeds, feed, fertilizer, etc.), compared to 1950."[9] Hold the applause, please. There is a very simple reason why they are generating more food. They are pumping the animals with antibiotics, arsenic, and ractopamine that make them grow faster, as well as using fillers in our feed products such as road-kill to curb costs.[10] That's right, animals that have been euthanized, slaughtered, or found by the side of the road are all fair game to be ground up and fed to animals produced for food. Animal waste, polyethylene plastic, and previously contaminated human food (such as food that has roach excrement on it) are all approved and used in animal feed. While the industry tries to pass this off as progress, it really comes down to cutting corners and producing cheap, unhealthy food products that are taking a disastrous toll on our environment and our health.

Let's review three of the most worrying additives to our meat and dairy products: the reckless use and abuse of antibiotics, the intentional feeding of arsenic to chickens and turkeys, and the not-so-wonder drug ractopamine given to pigs that comprise your bacon breakfast.

The End of Antibiotics

Think about the number of times we have used antibiotics to get back to our healthy, happy selves. What would happen if another swine flu hit? In 2009, swine flu reached near epidemic proportions, and twelve thousand Americans died.[11] Can you imagine a world where you can't recover from the flu? Sadly, this is a very real possibility, because we are giving factory-farm animals four-fifths of all the antibiotics produced.[12] In fact, in 2011, factory-farm animals received almost four times as many antibiotics as humans. The antibiotics are fed to the animals due to the filthy conditions in the factory farms, which are causing an antibiotic resistant epidemic. The CDC, USDA, and FDA all recognize and acknowledge that this overuse of antibiotics in our food supply is contributing to the antibiotic resistance that is becoming a significant threat to public health. Surprisingly, little is done to remediate this problem. In fact, more Americans die from antibiotic-resistant bacteria each year than from HIV/AIDS. The problem is that antibiotic use in our food is not declining but actually increasing. In 2011, more antibiotics were given to animals than ever before. We are rapidly reaching the end of the antibiotic era, placing us on the cusp of a monumental health crisis.

Why do cows, pigs, and chickens need antibiotics? The animals in factory farms are fed our antibiotics because horrendous factory farms produce prime conditions for disease. In order to keep the animals alive and to promote growth at a faster pace (from the growth hormones), animals are given therapeutic doses of antibiotics, so they can survive long enough to make it to slaughter. In other words, antibiotics are being used as preventative measures, rather than cures as they were intended.

Eighty percent of all the antibiotics manufactured in the United States are fed to the over twenty-seven billion animals raised for food each year.[13] An added and even ironic problem is that the animals do not even absorb the majority of the antibiotics. Animals only absorb about 15 to 20 percent of the antibiotics. The rest is excreted in their waste, which then contaminates our water and soil. This means we can pick up antibiotic-resistant bacteria from drinking water, swimming in a river, or eating food that has been fertilized with animal manure. No one is safe.

The antibiotics fed to the animals wouldn't be such a problem if they weren't the same antibiotics that we use to cure our illnesses. Alexander Fleming, who invented penicillin, warned that issuing non-lethal doses of an antibiotic makes the bacteria resistant. Substantial research reveals that exposure to low dosages of antibiotics like the ones given to animals causes enough stress on the bacteria to increase their rate of mutations. This process, called mutagenesis, is basically creating more virulent, hard-to-kill strains of bacteria that are resistant to drugs. These bacteria cause foodborne illnesses and problems such as urinary tract infections. In recent years, there has been a significant increase in UTIs, especially linked to the consumption of chicken. This isn't just a coincidence. Tests now show that bacteria continue to multiply in the presence of drugs designed to kill them.[14]

The overuse of antibiotics given to animals is now posing a major threat to human health, as bacteria is developing resistance faster than we could ever come up with new cures. Researchers are frantically pressing the government to act. Citing that antibiotics are the "crown jewels" of modern medicine, at a Congressional hearing the Director of the Center for Science in the Public Interest for food safety pleaded with Congress, "We must not continue to jeopardize the effectiveness of these drugs by using them recklessly for non-therapeutic uses on farms and in animal factories. Otherwise, consumers may face longer illnesses, more hospitalizations, and more fatalities when exposed to resistant strains of common foodborne pathogens."[15] Already the Infectious Diseases Society of America (IDSA) declared that antibiotic-resistant infections are an epidemic in the United States. Study after study is finding that the therapeutic dosage given to animals is costing lives. About two million people contract antibiotic-resistant infections, and ninety thousand per year are dying.[16] Yet the pharmaceutical and animal industries continue to deny the scientific evidence. This is despite the fact that the World Health Organization has also declared that the therapeutic use of antibiotics in farm animals contributes to the rise in antibiotic resistance. Friends, the science is crystal clear. Continuing down this path is a prescription for catastrophe.

Of particular concern are antibiotic-resistant, foodborne illnesses, caused by fecal contamination of meat. Recent studies show that 78 percent of our turkeys and 75 percent of our chickens contained antibiotic-resistant *salmonella*, and of the 95 percent of the chickens contaminated with tetracycline, half of them were antibiotic resistant.[17] All of these numbers are up since 2010.

Already we are experiencing nearly double the rate of hospitalizations from foodborne illnesses. For example, in Los Angeles in October 2013, there was a *salmonella* outbreak at the Foster Farms facility. Foster Farms is the tenth-largest chicken producer and banks between $1.9 and $2.3 billion per year.[18] Chickens are particularly susceptible to fecal contamination because their skin is left on for human consumption. However, what is concerning is the laissez-faire attitude toward this outbreak. Foster Farms had nearly a dozen reports in 2013 that found fecal contamination on their carcasses. The USDA contends that the rate of *salmonella* contamination at Foster Farms is on par with the rest of the chicken industry. Dan Englejohn, assistant administrator of the USDA's Office of Field Operation, states that "noncompliance is in no way indicative that there was a process out of control." Really, Mr. Englejohn? This viewpoint is cause for concern. Just because everyone is contaminating the food does not mean it is okay! Clearly we need to completely overhaul the regulatory system or, better yet, to avoid eating meat and dairy altogether.

Moreover, according to Caroline Smith DeWall, Food Safety Director for the Center for Science in the Public Interest, this new strain of *salmonella* at Foster Farms was more potent and was modified from antibiotic use.

Of those stricken, 42 percent were hospitalized. This rate is nearly *double* what we have seen in the past from foodborne-illness outbreaks and forecasts what we can expect to see if antibiotic use is not curtailed. On a comforting note, all of the chicken that was contaminated with fecal matter was stamped with the USDA-inspection mark of approval.[19]

Other lesser known pathogens, such as *Yersinia enterocolitica*, found in pigs, are also becoming antibiotic resistant and are becoming even more prominent in our grocery store products than other well-known foodborne illnesses. A recent Consumer Reports study found this bacterium in nearly 70 percent of all pig products from nationally recognized grocery stores.[20] Yersinia enterocolitica affects nearly one hundred thousand Americans each year. Of note is that Yersinia entercolitica is *not* one of the pathogens tested under the USDA HACCP plan. This means that even though it contaminates over half of the pig products sold in stores, the Department of Agriculture cannot require a recall. The plan is seen to be "meeting its goals." According to the USDA, "very low contamination levels in hog carcasses indicate that companies' practices are adequately controlling pathogens." This thinking seems a little flawed if we are not testing for all of the pathogens. We are essentially working off of plans that are doomed to fail the consumer because they are not comprehensive. Why are we not testing for all bacteria? Isn't our health more important? It's time we stop putting our health in severe jeopardy.

Harmful bacteria are finding ways into our kitchens. Some of the bacteria are so stuck to the meat that you can't even wash them off. Appetizing. But don't get too excited. When we wash off bacteria from animal carcasses in our kitchen sinks, the water can send bacteria flying up and onto dish towels, countertops, and other food products as far as three feet away. We've just increased our chances of contamination.

Physicians and national organizations are urging the FDA to remove antibiotics from our food. Due to the rising resistance, way back in June 2001, the American Medical Association passed a resolution that opposed non-therapeutic use of antibiotics for livestock production.[21] Guess what? The FDA chose to ignore this advice and continue to approve drugs. Recently the FDA approved the use of cefquinome despite protests from the American Medical Association and the CDC that this antibiotic comes from a class of medicines that is one of the last defenses against life-threatening, human diseases.[22]

What is confusing is that the FDA recognized back in 1977 that the therapeutic use of the three major drugs—penicillin, chlortetracycline, and oxytetracycline—it approved for use in farm animals was "not shown to be safe."[23] The FDA initiated the steps to withdraw these drugs when the agribusiness industry stepped up and lobbied Congress to halt the withdrawal process. Since then, the FDA has abandoned taking a stand for American health in favor of corporate interests and violated federal laws in the process.

However, in December 2013, the FDA announced new, voluntary regulatory guidelines to phase out growth enhancers in livestock over the next three years. The FDA finally acknowledged that administering the same antimicrobial drugs used in both humans and animals can contribute to resistance. Eli Lilly and Company and Zoetis, two of the largest drug makers, were asked to revise their labels and remove animal production as one of its acceptable uses. While this looks like a step in the right direction, the problem is with the word "voluntary." According to Congresswoman Louise Slaughter, the only microbiologist in Congress, the FDA's plan is "an inadequate response with no mechanisms for enforcement and no metric for success."[24] Congresswoman Slaughter, we have to wholeheartedly agree. Friends, let's be real. If producers are given the chance to "opt in" to a plan that might cost them money, do you really think they will happily oblige? It seems extremely doubtful at best. Looking at the FDA's history of issuing voluntary guidelines in 2012 that received little to no response, we can guess that these guidelines will receive a similar response.

Fortunately, not all of Congress is blind to the effects of abusing antibiotics and wants to stand on the sidelines while industries make antibiotics ineffective. Congresswoman Slaughter (NY) and Congressman Harris Waxman (CA) have both sponsored two new bills to curb antibiotic use and provide for better regulation. The Delivering Antimicrobial

Transparency in Animals Act and Preservation of Antibiotics for Medical Treatment Act both seek to actually regulate the use of antibiotics and enforce better usage and guidelines.[25] They would provide the FDA with a more substantive understanding of how antibiotics are being used and whether the FDA's voluntary program is effective. The Preservation of Antibiotics for Medical Treatment Act is widely supported among the medical community. Yet statistics indicate both bills only have about a 1 percent chance of being enacted. This is pathetic to say the least.

Think about the death toll when antibiotics no longer work. We are in a huge economic crisis, and yet we are spending between $4 and $5 billion dollars a year on antimicrobial resistance. This pales in comparison to the $45 billion the chicken industry alone rakes in every year.[26] Yet it doesn't pay for the external costs of its production. These health costs society has to bear will only increase if we continue down this path.[27] Already, pig farms are implicated in the rise of a new strain of MRSA, which is a potentially fatal disease and kills more people than AIDS per year.

Massive pandemics are on the horizon. However, the industry and our government are more inclined to protect corporate interests. USDA Secretary Tom Vilsack was quick to rename swine flu with the innocuous title H1N1. It's the same way the industry hides feces in our meat by calling it *E. coli* or *salmonella*. It is all about the marketing message and placing distance between the industry and its consequences. The USDA didn't hide its favorability for protecting the pork industry either. Mr. Vilsack stated during the 2009 swine flu outbreak that the USDA was doing "everything to ensure the hog industry was safe and sound."[28] No mention of the American public, despite the 250,000 Americans who were hospitalized. In the face of the World Health Organization issuing the highest pandemic level alert, the National Pork Producers Council stated that "[t]his flu is being called something it isn't . . . it is ruining people's lives."[29] The latter sentiment is one that we couldn't agree with more. The agribusiness industry and the USDA and FDA's continual backing of industry interests that promote antibiotic resistance are without a doubt ruining American lives, not to mention our pocketbooks. As antibiotic resistance is on the rise, this cost is only expected to increase as well. This is all preventable. It's time we reclaimed antibiotics and kept their integrity for curing illnesses intact.

Everything Is Not Better With Bacon

Ever heard of ractopamine? Most people haven't, but it is the main ingredient in the growth additive, Paylean, given to 80 percent of slaughtered pigs that then become our ham and bacon staples.[30] Ractopamine is a toxin that, as it warns on its label, is "not for human use." Clearly, this means we should not be ingesting any amount of this toxin. Yet as much as 20 percent of ractopamine residue can be found in the meat we eat. Although the drug manufacturer prides itself on the fact that this poison is tasteless, we find that information more terrifying than optimistic.

Ractopamine is given to pigs a few weeks before they are slaughtered to make the meat leaner and let the farmer get more bang for his buck. Since it gives higher feed efficiencies, it raises profits. While this works out nicely for farmers and the drug manufacturer, Elanco, a division of Eli Lilly and Company, the same benefits are not conferred on consumers or the animals. The FDA approved the use of ractopamine back in 1999 for use in pigs, and has since approved its use for beef cattle in 2003 and turkeys in 2008. However, ractopamine is not the wonder drug it is sold as.

Ractopamine belongs to the beta-agonists drug group, the opposite of beta blockers. Essentially, it mimics stress hormones and increases heart rate. Since its inception, the FDA has received over two hundred thousand reports of pigs that have adverse reactions, such as "hyperactivity, trembling, broken limbs, and inability to walk."[31] Imagine the unreported number. The label on the drug itself states that the product can cause "downer pigs," which are those too sick to move or get up. Common sense says that consuming an animal in this state is not healthy. The industry and its major producers that use ractopamine, such as Smithfield and Tyson, suggest that it is perfectly safe. The safety claims that the FDA based approval on for the drug, came from tests conducted by the manufacturer itself. Apparently they saw no blatant conflict of interest.

In case you were wondering, the FDA has not approved beta-agonists drugs for human use. It is surprising then that they set "tolerance" levels for ractopamine residues in our bacon, ham, and pulled-pork products. If a product is not for human use and is known to cause cardiovascular issues, we shouldn't be receiving any amount whatsoever. There should be a zero-tolerance policy.

Ractopamine is one of the most controversial growth-promoting drugs. About 160 countries have banned the drug due to its health consequences in pigs and known, negative impacts on the human cardiovascular system. Russia, which imported about $500 million worth of pork and beef products, banned US imports in 2012.[32] This did not go over well with the United States. Instead of re-evaluating the food-safety concerns Russia presented, the United States petitioned international CODEX standards and tried to gain widespread, global acceptance of ractopmaine. The United States claimed that Russia's move was not motivated by food-safety concerns but by financial protection of its own pork industry. It is apparently a very foreign concept for our government to understand why another government would restrict a toxin in the food system for safety reasons. Recently Russia lifted its ban on US products under the notion that upon testing, no ractopamine residues are found in imports.[33] The United States does very little testing for residues. In 2011, it simply didn't test about 22 billion pounds of pork produced. On the off chance that meat is tested for ractopamine, the toxin is frequently found. Think about this: if you ate pork that year, most likely it wasn't tested for this toxin.

The United States' actions are nothing short of depressing and horrifying. Ractopamine has been shown to cause heart damage, developmental defects, and fertility problems, in addition to extremely sick animals that are turned into food.[34] Why would our country that strives to be a model of opportunity, health, and prosperity knowingly compromise its citizens' health? We can't rely on industry and drug manufacturers to keep citizens' best interests at the forefront, because they only care about profits. We can do better than contaminated bacon. It's time we heeded the warning and steered clear of these "prized" meat products.

Arsenic, My Dear?

Some industry practices, such as the use of arsenic, cross the line of imprudence into insanity. In 2013, the FDA finally admitted that there is indeed arsenic added to our chicken and turkey. Before we get too excited about this news, know that the FDA has, for some reason, needed convincing to acknowledge the risks associated with this problem. For nearly five years, the FDA has chosen to ignore petitions filed against it for allowing arsenic use until now.[35]

Since the 1940s, chickens and other poultry have been given arsenic in their feed in order to make them grow faster and improve meat pigmentation. By 2010, about 88 percent of the nine billion chickens produced were fed arsenic.[36] The most common form of arsenic fed to chickens is called roxarsone, manufactured by the well-known pharmaceutical mogul, Pfizer. Roxarsone is an organic form of arsenic that is less toxic than its inorganic counterpart. For years, the poultry industry claimed that "there is no reason to believe that there are any human health hazards from this type of use."[37] The FDA sang a similar tune, claiming that there were no residues left in meat. Disturbingly, the industry and FDA are sorely wrong.

Let's look at Prairie Grove in Washington County, Arkansas, home of the poultry giant, Tyson, and its "100 percent All Natural" and "Kid Tested, Kid Approved" chicken. Prairie Grove is surrounded by chicken-factory farms where farmland is regularly spread with arsenic-laden litter. Prairie Grove's cancer rate is fifty times higher than the national average.[38] Similarly, in the Delmarva Peninsula that contains some of the biggest chicken-producing states, the cancer rates are alarmingly high, especially among young children. Why are the cancer rates so high? Arsenic doesn't just magically disappear once it is given to animals. It is either excreted in the manure that then makes its way into our environment or remains in the chicken that winds up on our grocery-store shelves. The air filters in the homes tested in Prairie Grove found arsenic levels exceeding even those in the soil outside. More than 350,000 tons of arsenic is applied to our land every year.[39] Clearly, arsenic in chicken production does have human-health effects.

Unlike the FDA, Johns Hopkins researchers undertook a landmark study in 2004 and 2013 to see if there was in fact arsenic residue in our meat.[40] The researchers tested not just the livers but the actual animal tissue, which is what consumers eat. They found arsenic residue in meat purchased from grocery stores across the nation.

Let's look at the findings from the most recent study that tested chicken, conducted in 2010 and 2011. The researchers compared organic chicken raised without arsenic and those they call "conventional," or what most people consume. They found that conventional chicken products had higher levels of arsenic in general and especially inorganic arsenic. Seventy percent of the samples contained inorganic arsenic that exceeded the FDA limits.[41] A bucket of fried chicken contained about fifty times the allowable arsenic than the "allowable" levels in a glass of water.

Although roxarsone is organic arsenic and supposedly less dangerous, these studies show that some of the arsenic is converted into the inorganic, toxic form from the bacteria inside chickens' guts. The EPA found that 65 percent of the arsenic in chicken meat converts to the inorganic form.[42] The organic arsenic also changes to inorganic when it is excreted in the waste and then distributed onto the field as part of the fertilizer.

While many other studies have shown the levels of arsenic to be below the FDA limits, no exposure to arsenic is good exposure. Arsenic is linked to a variety of health problems, namely cancer, but also cognitive defects; cardiovascular, immune, and endocrine problems; partial paralysis; miscarriages; and type 2 diabetes.[43] Why are we allowing an unnecessary public-health threat when we can choose to eliminate the problem?

The FDA suspended roxarsone in 2011 after these findings showed the level of poisonous, inorganic arsenic in chickens, but it never banned the drug. Finally, in 2013, the FDA ordered three of the four drugs to be removed from the market. The makers Zoetis and Fleming, subsidies of Pfizer, voluntarily pulled these three drugs in 2011 after the findings of inorganic arsenic. Why the FDA has been dragging its feet when it comes to with drawing arsenic in the animal's feed that remains in our food is a mystery. Even the makers of the drugs pulled them from the market before the FDA did.[44] It has taken the FDA over fifty years to act somewhat in the public interest. One version of organic arsenic, nitrasone, which is mainly used in turkeys, is still on the market.[45] This could be a reason to rethink our Thanksgiving menu.

Americans eat more chicken and poultry than any other type of meat—about eighty-three pounds per American in 2011.[46] Chicken is marketed as the "healthiest" and leanest meat. Somehow eating arsenic doesn't translate to health. This practice is beyond irresponsible. We should never let ourselves or corporations play chicken with our health.

Deadly Dioxins

Although not added to our food products, the presence of dioxins in our food is not new. Since 1994, the Environmental Protection Agency (EPA) declared dioxins a serious health threat and some of the most deadly and harmful chemicals known to science. Dioxins are a group of chemicals in our environment that are formed from the by-product of processes such as herbicide manufacturing. However, what most people don't know is that today between 93 percent and 96 percent of human exposure to dioxins comes from eating meat and dairy products. Twenty-three percent of dioxin exposure comes from milk and dairy alone. The highest levels of dioxins are found in beef products, then dairy, milk, chicken, pork, fish, and eggs.[47] Dioxins are known for causing health problems, such as cancer, damage to the immune system, and developmental problems as in birth defects as well as fertility issues, endometriosis, diabetes, lung and respiratory problems, skin disorders, and for men, lowered testosterone levels.

Humans are particularly susceptible to high concentrations of dioxins because the chemicals bioaccumulate in animals' fat up the food chain. The animals can be exposed to dioxins through the pesticides and herbicides in their feed as well as pollutants in factory farms. Dioxins are fat soluble, meaning they are stored in the fatty tissue of the animals. Similarly, the dioxins accumulate in our fat. Problematically, men have no mechanism for getting rid of dioxins, and the only way women can lower their level of dioxins is by passing on the toxins to their babies either via umbilical cords or through breastfeeding. Obviously, these aren't great options, as this sets up your child for health problems. Studies indicate that many babies are born already pre-polluted with carcinogens from their umbilical cords.

Although the FDA loves to set acceptable thresholds and tolerance limits on toxins, the EPA confirms that there is no safe level of exposure. More worrisome, there is no safe threshold below which dioxins will not cause cancer. What this means, friends, is that *any exposure can instigate cancer growth*. In July 2002, a study found a direct association between dioxin exposure and increased risk of breast cancer. As dioxins are by-products and not intentionally manufactured, many organizations collectively agree that dioxin exposure can best be avoided by not eating meat and dairy products.[48] It really is that simple.

After acknowledging that dioxins are known carcinogens, it would seem that the EPA would act expeditiously to monitor our exposure and set regulations. However, the EPA has consecutively and continuously missed its own deadlines for releasing its newest study on dioxins. In the meantime, the Dairy Association and National Chicken Council, among other pharmaceutical and Big Ag groups, are vehemently lobbying against releasing the report. They have repeatedly urged the White House to block the EPA study.[49] Even the FDA urges consumers not to "avoid any particular foods because of dioxins."[50] Did the FDA miss the memo stating dioxins are cancer causing and most of our exposure comes from milk and meat products?

We should be allowed access to information on toxins that could lead to a potentially fatal illness and be told the warnings associated with eating animal products. Big Ag and many drug manufacturers would rather distort the truth about the dangers of dioxins in our meat and dairy products than stand to lose profits. This is shameful when we know that dioxins are referred to as "the most toxic chemicals known to science."[51] We are hoping the EPA doesn't cave to industry dollars and interests but rather takes a stand and lives up to the "protection" part of its title.

False Security Propaganda

The FDA proclaims that "the US food supply is among the safest and most nutritious in the world."[52] Knowing the amount of toxic chemicals in our food and the government's push to continue to use unsafe chemicals, it seems quite a stretch to use the words "safest" and "most nutritious" in connection with our food system. America, this is why our food system is broken. We have agencies promoting a false sense of safety and security. Realistically, our food system falls very short of this idealistic statement. It's time we take our food system into our own hands and push the government to live up to this sentiment.

Know your Sh!t Solutions:

1) *Read nutritional labels. If you can't pronounce the ingredients, don't buy the food products.*
2) *Be aware that all the ingredients may not be listed, so eat at your own risk. Anything that says "natural" or "artificial" flavoring is probably not something you should be ingesting. Think bleach and rocket fuel.*
3) *Buy organic as much as possible.*
4) *Don't play around with your health. You only have one body, and you have to treat it right. Avoid all animal products, especially factory-farmed products, as much as possible.*

CHAPTER 5

A Hamburger Seasoned with Feces, Please!

We are getting more than just fries with our meals. We are eating sh!t. We are not talking about just unhealthy food but actual, animal feces. As former USDA meat-inspector David Carney aptly stated, "We used to trim the sh!t off the meat . . . then we washed the sh!t off the meat . . . now the consumer eats the sh!t off the meat."[1]

Although most Americans don't think about eating feces in their food, eating sh!t is a well-known national problem. Most of us have heard of *salmonella, E. coli,* and the less well-known *Campylobacter* and *Listeria.* These names don't scare us because they are so often thrown around with the high level of outbreaks and recalls each year. Even restaurant menus warn us about the potential for disease by emphasizing the necessity of cooking meat to a desired temperature to avoid foodborne illnesses.

Most of us think of *salmonella* and *E. coli* as just some stomach bugs, but we are not aware that these are the actual scientific names for the bacteria in animal feces. Every time you see *E. coli, salmonella,* or *Campylobacter,* read it as animal sh!t. This is why we get sick from eating raw cookie dough or spinach that has been doused with animal crap from factory farms. Disgusting but true: our food is tainted with animal feces that comes from our sloppy-but-accepted farming conditions and laser-fast slaughtering practices that have little oversight from government agencies.

Researchers at the University of Maryland randomly sampled two hundred packages of ground meat in Washington, D.C.-area grocery stores. The researchers found that 6 percent of beef, 35 percent of chicken, 24 percent of turkey, and 16 percent of pork were contaminated with *salmonella.* Eighty-four percent of these *salmonella* strains were antibiotic resistant.[2] Shockingly, the most recent Consumer Reports study made headlines as it found 97 percent of chicken sold in retail-grocery stores were contaminated with *salmonella*—half of which contained multi-resistant strains to antibiotics.

The food industry and agribusiness try to disassociate *E. coli* and *salmonella* from its true identity by using their scientific names. The industry is trying to make conversation about feces in your meat seem normal and commonplace. We should not be making light of this problem. We can all agree there is nothing normal about eating sh!t. Even more egregious is that the industry tries to pass the blame for foodborne illness onto the consumer for not cooking the meat at high temperatures. According to one industry spokesperson,

> "The consumer has the most responsibility but refuses to accept it. Raw meats are not idiot-proof. They can be mishandled and when they are, it's like handling a hand grenade. If you pull the pin, somebody's going to get hurt."

Firstly, why is it okay to sell potential food grenades in our grocery stores? Admitting that these foods are potentially dangerous makes the blame-the-victim response completely unfair. Even Patricia Griffin, the Chief of the Enteric Diseases Epidemiology Branch at the Centers for Disease Control, had a problem with this industry attitude, stating, "Is it reasonable that if a consumer undercooks a hamburger . . . their three-year-old dies?" Tell that to all the mothers and fathers who have lost their children to burgers that were not cooked at perfect temperatures.

However, this blame game is more than unfair—it is also completely wrong. Researchers found that infants and toddlers sitting near raw meat in grocery carts had an increased risk of *salmonella* or *Campylobacter* infection.[3] Studies looking at the direct correlation between drug-resistant urinary tract infections and consuming contaminated chicken found that one doesn't even have to eat the chicken to become contaminated.[4] That's right. Merely handling the contaminated chicken was enough to cause infection. It seems like the meat industry is a little too quick to place blame on the consumer. If just being in the proximity of raw meat increases our infection chances, then how is cooking going to help?

So what happens when we cook chicken? Studies found that when we brought chicken into our homes and cooked with it, fecal contamination was found on everything from utensils to countertops and aprons. Remarkably, even after everything was bleached and washed thoroughly, antibiotic-resistant pathogens were still alive and well. A University of Arizona study confirmed that in an omnivore's house, the kitchen sink is dirtier than the toilet bowl, meaning there is more crap in our kitchen than where we go to take a crap. Really, think about that again. Our meat is more tainted than a toilet bowl.

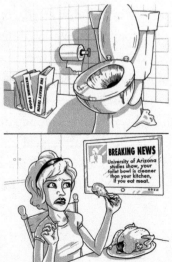

How can we avoid this issue? The researchers concluded that the only way is to not buy chicken. The carcasses are so contaminated that any chicken is bound to pose a threat. If the industry really wants to warn the consumer, shouldn't food and restaurant menus state: "Warning: You might ingest animal feces with this steak"? Now that warning might actually produce a reaction.

More than just plain disgusting, the prevalence of feces in our food products is a serious threat to our health. Eating sh!t can (and does) kill us. Today, forty-eight million Americans, about one in every six people each year, are affected by foodborne illnesses. Friends, this is about one-third of America. *Salmonella* poisoning alone affects one million Americans each year. A scary realization is that these statistics underestimate the number of people who are affected, because the Centers for Disease Control (CDC) and World Health Organization (WHO) never know the true extent of outbreaks. Although fortunately the number of deaths is much smaller than the number infected—about three thousand die each year—there shouldn't be any reason for us to be getting sick from feces, let alone die from eating it. Beyond the three thousand recorded people who died last year from eating feces, thousands of others are now living with malfunctioning organs. Eating crap can permanently wreck our bodies.

Dying from Dinner

Six months after graduating from kindergarten, six-year-old Alex Donley ate a hamburger and died four days later without a single functioning organ. The toxins produced by *E. coli* had turned Alex's organs to mush, including entire parts of his brain.[5] Nancy Donley, Alex's mother, had to watch helplessly as her son suffered from abdominal cramps and severe diarrhea, to the point that he was wearing bloody diapers when his bowels became uncontrollable. Alex lost neurological control and experienced hallucinations and collapsed lungs all within a few days. Alex died unable to recognize his mother and father, all because he unknowingly ate sh!t that was in his burger.

Three-year-old Brianne suffered a similar fate. Brianne's mother watched as

> "Her intestines swelled to three times their normal size and she was placed on a ventilator. Emergency surgery became essential and her colon was removed. Her heart was so swollen it was like a sponge and bled from every pore. Her liver and pancreas shut down and she was gripped by thousands of convulsions, which caused blood clots in her eyes. We were told she was brain dead."[6]

Sadly, Alex and Brianne's stories are a snapshot of the heartache from what the CDC calls a *preventable* illness.

Let us get a few points straight about food poisoning and foodborne illness. It is more than just stomach bugs and twenty-four-hour diarrhea. As Alex and Brianne's stories attest, foodborne illnesses can cause serious and severe complications such as hemorrhagic colitis, bloodstream infection, meningitis, joint infection, kidney failure, paralysis, miscarriage, and arthritis.[7] *E. coli* can literally melt your insides and *Campylobacter* can produce acute paralysis that results in a premature death.

Young children are especially susceptible to health complications. For example, *E. coli O157:H7* is the leading cause of acute kidney failure, or hemolytic-uremic syndrome (HUS), in children and babies. The frightening aspect of HUS is that there isn't a cure. Doctors can tend to the symptoms but, along with the parents, they are virtually helpless to stop the infection from spreading. For the lucky ones who do survive, most of these children have to live with dialyses for the rest of their lives.

Let's be honest, we wouldn't knowingly eat animal sh!t. Why are we not aware that we are eating feces and that fecal contamination is ubiquitous?

What's the Beef with E. coli?

E. coli made headlines in 1993 from the Jack in the Box fiasco, where hundreds of people across the nation fell ill and four died from eating undercooked hamburgers. Before this notorious incident, talk of food-borne pathogens was infrequent, if it occurred at all. However, the Jack in the Box incident pushed foodborne illnesses, as well as the glaring gaps in our food safety system, into the spotlight. The current food-safety policy was extremely lax. Inspectors from the USDA Food Safety and Inspection Service (FSIS) followed a "poke and sniff" method where they merely looked at the carcasses to see if there was contamination.[8] This look-and-see method dates back to the first Federal Meat Inspection Act of 1906. Yet meat production as we know it had changed significantly in both the production of more meat and the less than sanitary conditions.

What was the government's response? FSIS declared *E. coli* an adulterant, which made it illegal to sell *E. coli*-contaminated meat. This means that processing plants had to start actually testing the meat. While the government's actions were praised, the meat industry had a very different response. In fact, it sued the government, claiming the USDA didn't have the authority to declare *E. coli* an adulterant and illegal to sell. We aren't quite sure what role they thought the USDA is reputed to have when it comes to food safety. Fortunately, a judge also didn't buy into the beef industry's ridiculous logic and declared in *Texas Food Industry Association v. Espy* that the USDA does, in fact, have the authority to make our food supply safer.[9] We know this seems like common sense, but the beef industry seemed to have a hard time swallowing this logic.

Interestingly, only one offending strand, *E. coli O157:H7*, was declared an adulterant in ground beef at the time. It took until 2012, almost twenty years later, for the FSIS to declare *E. coli* an adulterant in beef trimmings as well as non-intact beef. It also took thousands of children and adults dying horrendous deaths for the USDA to declare six more strands of *E. coli* adulterants. It took another two years after several hundred more Americans were stricken with a virulent form of *E. coli* for the Obama administration to declare these six strands adulterants as well.[10] We know government can be slow moving, but this crawl toward a common-sense ruling is beyond frustrating.

Even though *E. coli* is naturally produced in the stomach linings of both humans and animals, there are about one hundred strains that are lethal. Many of these strains are now antibiotic resistant due to antibiotic-overuse in factory farms. *E. coli*, by nature, is extremely resilient. It can live on kitchen countertops for days, it can withstand freezing temperatures, and it can survive heat of up to 160 degrees Fahrenheit. Unlike *salmonella* poisoning, which requires a fairly large dose of the pathogen, it only takes as few as five to ten *E. coli* particles to infect you. This means a microscopic piece of hamburger meat can prove fatal.

For those who do survive the illness, recent studies indicate that *E. coli* has frighteningly long-term health effects. For instance, in May 2000, heavy rain caused manure runoff from factory farms to enter the nearby waterway and aquifer that supplied the drinking water for a town in Ontario. Five thousand people were sickened after drinking the contaminated tap water. The long-term study published in 2010 on this incident found that those sickened "had a 33 percent greater likelihood of developing high blood pressure, a 210 percent greater risk of heart attack or stroke, and a 340 percent greater risk of kidney problems in the eight years following the outbreak."[11] The study found that everyone, no matter their level of infection, had an increased risk of long-term health problems.

Studies consistently find that lifelong-health complications include higher incidence of heart attack and stroke, continuous digestive problems, onset of arthritis, permanent brain damage, end-stage kidney disease, and insulin-dependent diabetes. These long-term consequences indicate a new side of foodborne illnesses that we haven't considered, because news stories tend to focus on immediate deaths and illnesses.

We have drastically underestimated the costs of foodborne illness to society. Our government's slow regulatory process shows obvious weaknesses in our food-safety system. Even more eye-opening is that *E. coli* is the most-regulated pathogen and the only pathogen declared an illegal adulterant.

This could be due to the fact that the industry's attitude has not shifted in more than twenty years. James Hodges, the vice president of the

American Meat Institute, declared, "The USDA will spend millions of dollars testing for these strains instead of using those limited resources toward preventive strategies that are far more effective in ensuring food safety."[12] Mr. Hodges, you are right. Prevention is key to mitigating food-borne illness. But, Mr. Hodges, what does the industry consider preventative? Surely it isn't starting to regulate the foul practices at factory farms that create this massive quantity of unregulated manure or avoiding eating the meat altogether as a wholesome preventative strategy. We are still waiting for a clear answer.

Ladies, Feeling the Burn Isn't Worth it

Ever had that uncomfortable burning sensation down in your privates? You constantly have to run to the restroom and are so uncomfortable and sore you just have no idea where to put yourself. Urinary tract infections affect millions of women each year, but they are not just from sex or hygiene. Increasingly, they are from eating chicken.

We tend to focus on the intestinal *E. coli* found in hamburgers, but there are strains of *E. coli* that cause extra-intestinal infections. This form of *E. coli* is becoming a huge problem and being cited as an "underappreciated killer."[13] *According to renowned physician Dr. Michael Greger, one strain of E. coli can cause urinary tract infections that infect the bloodstream and cause up to thirty-six thousand deaths per year.*

How do we know it's in the chicken? Well, researchers spent billions of health-care dollars testing nearly two thousand food samples. They found that half of retail poultry samples were contaminated with the UTI-associated strains of *E. coli*. Ladies, when we eat contaminated chicken, it infects our lower intestinal tracts, and the infection creeps into our bladders, causing us that immensely painful illness. UTIs are serious business. Beyond the burn, they have the potential to invade the bloodstream and cause sepsis or blood poisoning, which can be fatal.

Researchers find that overcrowding in factory farms, especially the confinement of egg-laying hens to small cages, is one of the premier risk factors for the disease in chickens called colibacillosis. More space would drastically reduce the most common disease in poultry by 33 percent. Remember, a chicken lives in a space smaller than the size of a piece of paper. The need to address this issue is paramount, as many of the UTIs from poultry are resistant to our most powerful remedies.[14]

How Clean is Our Salmonella-Tainted Chicken and Turkey?

How many times have we eaten raw cookie dough and joked about *salmonella* poisoning? While chicken is touted as the healthiest meat, it is also the most feces-contaminated meat on the market. A breaking news study by Consumer Reports found that 97 percent of the chicken sold is covered in fecal contamination. This means it is extremely hard or nearly impossible to eat feces-free chicken. What's more is that half of these chickens contained antibiotic-resistant pathogens.

This finding wouldn't be such a problem if chicken consumption was relatively minimal, but chicken is the most consumed meat product in America. Americans ate about 100 million pounds in wings alone during the Super Bowl. That's one day and 1.25 billion chicken wings.[15] While red-meat consumption has been slightly decreasing over the past few years, chicken consumption is at an all-time high and only expected to increase. Chicken prices have not only fallen, but the meat is also touted as our "leanest" meat. At a time when our health is failing and our waistlines are expanding, the lean-meat myth is rapidly increasing chicken consumption. Our indulgence in chicken mirrors the rapid increase in *salmonella* outbreaks. Coincidence? We think not.

While *E. coli* is often the most talked-about foodborne pathogen, *salmonella* kills more Americans than any other foodborne pathogen and is increasingly the most common. *Salmonella* poisoning is now responsible for about one million infections due to the increase in outbreaks. Recent studies indicate that up to half of the chickens, turkeys, and eggs found in our grocery stores are contaminated. Unlike *E. coli*, which has only about one hundred strains, *salmonella* has about 2,500 different, lethal strains. These strains are virulent by nature. Cooking your eggs sunny-side up, scrambled, or over-easy does not kill *salmonella,* according to studies by the American Egg Board.

In 2011 alone, there were nine *salmonella* outbreaks.[16] There were also nine *salmonella* outbreaks in 2010, and they weren't small either. One of the 2010 outbreaks led to a recall of half a billion eggs.[17] One of the latest outbreaks on September 29, 2011, which infected about 129 people in thirty-four different states, was antibiotic resistant.[18] This is compared to 2006, when there was only one major *salmonella* outbreak.

The increase in *salmonella* outbreaks is directly attributable to the increase in consumption of poultry products as well as factory farm conditions and practices.[19] Before eggs were produced in factory farms, *salmonella* in eggs was virtually nonexistent. Now, *salmonella*-tainted eggs infect nearly two hundred thousand Americans every year. Keeping over one hundred thousand chickens in cramped conditions with massive amounts of fecal-airborne dust rapidly increases the spread of *salmonella.* Additionally, CDC researchers found that more than one million cases of *salmonella* poisoning are directly linked to the practice of feeding ground-up animals to other animals.[20] Once hens can no longer lay any more eggs, they are ground up and used as additives to chicken feed. Studies indicate that over half of the chicken feed given to factory-farmed chickens contains *salmonella.*

The increase in *salmonella* is becoming an increasing health cost to society. Like *E. coli,* studies indicate that *salmonella* can also cause long-term health effects, such as continuous and persistent irritable bowel syndrome. *Salmonella* can also start as food poisoning and leave the unknowing consumer with reactive arthritis, which is a chronic and permanent, debilitating form of arthritis.[21]

European countries have declared it illegal to sell *salmonella*-tainted meat. This could be why Europe boasts such a low rate of contamination. Similarly, since the United States declared *E. coli* an adulterant, its prevalence has decreased by about 30 percent.[22]

However, *salmonella* poisoning is still not illegal. That's right. It is legal to sell *salmonella*-tainted meat. While only 65 percent of meat is contaminated with *E. coli*, about 80 percent to 97 percent of poultry is contaminated with *salmonella*.[23] The most recent Foster Farms *salmonella* outbreak in 2013 that sickened over five hundred people glaringly shows that *salmonella* outbreaks are on the rise and there is a drastic need for reform.[24]

One would think the USDA would respond to this growing concern and also make *salmonella* illegal. Making it illegal to sell meat that could cripple and kill our children is apparently a hard concept for the USDA to grasp. Instead, the USDA has chosen to throw its hands in the air and claim that "there are numerous sources of contamination which might contribute to the overall problem." According to them, it is "unjustified to single out the meat industry and ask that the Department require it to identify its raw products as being hazardous to health."[25,26] With this logic, we would never put warning labels on anything that has another, albeit far-fetched, possibility of laying claim to responsibility.

To the USDA's credit, they did try to regulate *salmonella* in the past. For example, in 1999 the USDA shut down a Supreme Beef plant in Texas. The plant had failed USDA testing three times, and as much as 45 percent of its meat was contaminated. The meat from Supreme Beef made up almost half of the national school lunch program. When the USDA shut the plant down, Supreme Beef challenged the decision, arguing that "*salmonella* shouldn't be regarded as an adulterant of ground beef."[27] Its argument was that since *salmonella* is so commonly found in food, it isn't an adulterant and should be considered normal. Essentially, since the meat corporations have contaminated their meat and do not take measures to prevent this, the frequent and consistent contamination means that our meat isn't tainted and we need to accept this as normal. Are they kidding?

Shockingly, the Appeals court upheld the decision that the USDA could *not* shut down a plant for contamination. The powerful meat industries have made it possible to legally sell contaminated meat.

So what's the real reason that the industries oppose regulation and we don't have policies to declare *salmonella* as illegal? Apparently it's too expensive to sell meat not covered in feces. We aren't kidding. That's the real reason. According to one industry spokesperson, "To get to zero is a real challenge . . . If we did nothing but testing for *salmonella* and non-0157s, there wouldn't be anything left to eat."[28] Others claim, "It's virtually impossible to have zero *salmonella,* according to the large-scale production conditions used here in the U.S., which help keep the price of poultry down. If you want chicken with no *salmonella*, it's going to cost a lot more money to produce."[29] Who else is game for paying more money for a better-quality product?

For any other industry, these answers would be wholly unacceptable. Imagine if car companies said it was too expensive to add seat belts to their cars, so we should all drive at our own risk. Or what if airlines said it was just too expensive to check and make sure that all of the equipment was functioning properly before takeoff? We wouldn't stand for it. We would either find alternative transportation or demand change. America, why are we not fighting for the same rights with our food?

Campylobacter is Paralyzing

Campylobacter is one of the most common foodborne pathogens, causing 2.5 million illnesses and costing the United States over one billion dollars in medical costs and lost productivity per year. Similar to *salmonella*, *Campylobacter* is typically found on chicken carcasses, as it is produced in the stomach linings of warm-blooded birds and some mammals. Studies have found that between 68 percent and 88 percent of chickens sold in grocery stores were contaminated with *Campylobacter. Campylobacter* is easily transmitted, as it only takes about five hundred bacterium or one tiny drop of chicken juice to cause infection. It can also survive in water and dairy lagoons.

While *Campylobacter* is not as fatal as *E. coli* can be, it is most serious when it affects children. It affects children twice as much as adults and can cause Guillain-Barré syndrome, an autoimmune reaction that can result in acute, permanent paralysis and even death. Guillain-Barré syndrome is like multiple sclerosis on speed—instead of taking years to cripple you, it takes a matter of days. Infection can start in a matter of hours after consumption. First, you start to lose feeling in your hands and feet. Then suddenly you can't walk, talk, or move. Next, you can't breathe and have to be put on a ventilator. Although Guillain-Barré syndrome generally runs a two-week course, it can leave its victim with lifelong disabilities or prove fatal if not caught in time. As many as 40 percent of *Campylobacter* cases lead to Guillain-Barré syndrome.[30] Why play Russian roulette with our health? With the amount of chicken that Americans consume weekly, we are increasing our chances of being struck down by one of these diseases when our luck runs out.

These Feed Ingredients Make Us Crazy

There are two ways sh!t gets into your meat and poultry: through the animal-feed ingredients and through lax standards in slaughterhouses and unsanitary conditions where the animals are raised.

Food-safety issues are related to how animals are raised as well as what they are fed. The animals you eat and drink milk from are being fed the waste of up to two hundred other dead animals. Using manure in feed is a type of "recycling" process to get rid of the excessive amount of manure.[31] Cows are fed chicken litter that is known to have residues of arsenic, antibiotics, and parasites such as tapeworms, *salmonella*, and *Campylobacter*.

The list of approved ingredients in feed is anything but a natural diet that cows, pigs, and chickens should be eating. These ingredients include: grains; massive amounts of pesticides; herbicides and insecticides used to produce the grain; by-products of slaughtered animals, which include unborn calf carcasses; by-products of dead animals (roadkill, euthanized animals, blood meal, diseased animals); animal fat and tallow; contaminated and adulterated food waste or food not fit for human consumption; antibiotics; drugs, such as arsenic in chickens; added minerals; and, last but not least, animal manure from other animals. The FDA also allows downed (meaning too sick to walk) and diseased animals to be slaughtered and fed to others.

While the FDA decides if feed ingredients are safe or not, it is clear that allowing feces as well as the remains of rotting, dead animals into meat is never safe. You don't need a government authority to tell you that this is a health risk. This practice only leads to disaster.

Mad cow disease is one dire example. It is produced when animals are forced to be carnivorous and eat the remains of other dead animals. While the European countries banned these practices, the FDA still allows chickens and pigs to eat rendered animal parts as well as blood products that can be infected with bovine spongiform encephalopathy, or mad cow disease. The FDA continues to allow this practice even after the first case of mad cow disease appeared in America in 2003 and the most recent case was reported in April 2012.[32]

As consumers, we assume that our governmental organizations are doing everything possible to warn consumers of possible infection and even take steps to prevent mad cow disease and other infections. While this disease is hard to detect and can have an incubation period of eight to ten years, the USDA doesn't find it worthwhile to test for mad cow disease. The USDA only tests about one-tenth of the cows slaughtered and imported for this brain-degenerative disease. An Arkansas court even banned meatpacker tests for mad cow disease—supporting the USDA's refusal to sell mad cow disease testing kits to an Arkansas meat-packer who wanted to test every one of his cows to assure his consumers that his meat was safe.[33] Can you imagine the government not allowing one packing company to test each and every cow! What could possibly motivate such blatant oversight? Could it be that the USDA is not concerned with what is best for public health and animals but rather fearful of having to test all cows and discovering more problems than it wants to deal with?

Packing Our Food with Feces

A government official, who chooses to remain anonymous, stated that a modern feedlot is akin to the crowded conditions during the Middle Ages in Europe where raw sewage ran down the streets.[34] Animals are frequently eating their meals while standing knee-deep in their own feces and urine. Pathogens such as *E. coli, Campylobacter,* and *salmonella* are produced in the animals' digestive systems and stomach linings and then excreted in manure and feces. Since foodborne illnesses are passed in manure, the cramped, filthy, stench-ridden, and inhumane conditions in factory farms and on feedlots are killing people and animals along with destroying ecosystems. With these conditions, combined with the lightning-fast pace of slaughterhouses that do not allow for proper cleaning and killing, it is no surprise that feces gets into meat products.

Since cows, pigs, and chickens live in their own waste, they arrive at the slaughterhouses caked in feces. This makes for easy pathogen transfer of *E. coli*, which can live in manure for up to ninety days.[35]

The pace of killing in the slaughterhouse is laser fast and extreme. As many as three hundred chickens are slaughtered per second. One cow is killed every twelve seconds. Think about how many cows died as you have read this chapter. There is no time to trim the sh!t off of the meat, let alone take the time to make sure there isn't cross-contamination between the pulled-out guts of a sick cow and those of a healthy cow.

Two tasks that can contribute to the most feces in your meat are the removal of hides caked in manure and the removal of the animal's digestive system, where pathogens are produced. As cows and pigs swing in the air from one foot, machines strip the feces-covered hides away from the animals. Yet at the breakneck pace, manure can fly. It can remain on the carcasses or be flung to other carcasses.

Second, the "gutting" table can contaminate the meat supply with pathogens when guts spill everywhere. One worker is expected to gut about sixty cows an hour. During Eric Schlosser's investigation for his bestselling book, *Fast Food Nation,* he found that gutting requires skill; it can take workers up to six months to learn how to pull out the guts and tie the intestines without spilling manure everywhere. Even when workers acquire this skill, Schlosser found that workers could only gut about two hundred consecutive cattle without spillage. As slaughterhouse workers have a 100 percent annual turnover rate, the prospect of gutting without spilling is not high. One IBP slaughterhouse in Lexington, Nebraska, reported that the hourly spillage rate of guts and manure was about 20 percent or every one in five carcasses.[36] Not good enough, friends.

If spilling guts isn't bad enough, the rate of contamination that makes its way to your kitchen counter is amplified by the lack of clean utensils used to cut the animals apart. One knife can contaminate literally hundreds of carcasses.

E. coli is more prevalent during the summer months, infecting about 50 percent of animals on feedlots compared to 1 percent during the winter. It is safe to assume that between one in every four animals infected with *E. coli* are killed at a slaughterhouse every hour. One animal infected with pathogens can contaminate about thirty-two thousand pounds of meat. Contrary to popular belief, your hamburger is not made from one cow but the meat from between forty to one hundred different cows. This is not a very comforting thought.

Centralizing Contamination

Food recalls are a direct indication that our food is contaminated. In fact, foodborne illness was ranked as the number-eight productivity killer in the United States.[37] A simple Google search indicates that there is a high level of contamination, as not a month goes by without some sort of meat, dairy, peanut, fruit, or egg recall due to foodborne pathogens.

To be perfectly clear, spinach and tomatoes do not produce *E. coli* or *salmonella*. When the media alarms us with recalls of spinach, tomatoes, cantaloupe, or even peanut butter, it is because pathogens from untreated manure used as fertilizer or spilled from factory farms and slaughterhouse waste have made their way into those food supplies.

The problem is that most of the food is not sent back to the plant, because contaminated food is only found out after the fact. When an outbreak happens, it can take months to discover the source, because of the lack of testing and oversight. Surprisingly, the USDA is not required to disclose where the tainted meat comes from in order to protect the corporations' reputations. The USDA cannot even disclose exactly to which supermarkets the meat was shipped. According to the meat corporations, disclosing where the tainted food products are sold is proprietary information and could harm their companies.

Even more shocking than this protect-the-corporation mindset is that the USDA has zero authority to initiate a recall of food. For years, the only authority the USDA and FDA had was to politely ask the company with said contaminated product to recall it. How can our government agencies that regulate our food do their job if they have zero enforcement policies? This is akin to a police officer asking a drunk driver to kindly turn himself or herself in to the station without having any legal right to arrest the drunk driver. This is the same public tragedy. The FDA, however, just gained the right to recall food with the passage of the Food Safety Modernization Act in 2010. The USDA has still not received the same authorization.

For years, researchers and scientists have warned that our meat production and slaughter system creates an ideal environment to spread the next big pandemic that will wipe out massive populations. Today the risk for contamination is magnified, as meat and dairy production is largely controlled by a few corporations that ship their products across the nation. When you combine this centralization, feed additives, cramped conditions at factory farms, and quick pace at the slaughterhouses with lax conditions, you have a recipe for disaster and sh!t in your food.

Learning from the Past? Not with HACCP or HIMP

The slaughterhouse conditions today are reminiscent of the famous muck-raking book, *The Jungle,* by Upton Sinclair, which prompted the Pure Food and Drug Act and Meat Inspection Act of 1906 to clean up the sickening conditions in slaughterhouses and meat-processing plants. While there might not be rats running around today, there sure as hell is manure flying.

Yet, since the passage of this act, Congress has done little, if anything, to pass laws that better regulate our food supply. In the time of President Roosevelt's presidency, 190 measures were proposed to regulate food safety. In the past decade, there has only been a handful of significant pieces of legislation introduced. To put this in perspective, the poultry industry today slaughters more birds in one day than it did during the entire year of 1930, and we have almost the same level of legislation.[38]

Back in 1998, the USDA opted to allow the corporations to regulate themselves and report their own cases of foodborne outbreaks under the Hazard Analysis and Critical Control Point (HACCP) program.[39] By adopting HACCP, corporations are assumed to be producing safe food. The USDA's seal of approval is applied to our food products *without* inspection. The public was never given the memo of this change. The Government Accountability Office, the investigative arm of Congress, has issued numerous reports over the years stating that the USDA's and FSIS's lack of adequate oversight and prevention of foodborne illnesses. The USDA has continuously not reported when a company fails to meet their HACCP plan requirements.[40] In one district, an FSIS inspector did not issue noncompliance reports for all fifteen of the plants that had violations. FSIS inspectors do not even ensure that the companies' HACCP plans are based on sound science.

Yet the USDA is moving in a worrying direction toward even more lax standards with their HIMP, or HACCP-Based Inspection Models Project. This policy would not only increase chicken speed lines by as much as 25 percent, but also replace USDA staff with employees from the processing plants. According to the USDA, this will better bolster *salmonella* detection.[41] Who are they kidding? This would mean that ten thousand chickens and turkeys would be processed per hour and overseen by a corporate employee. No one can look at and inspect up to ninety chickens a minute. It is simply impossible. Not to mention under the new guidelines, the employees can only see the backs of the chickens, not the fronts, which are the breast meat.[42]

A former USDA poultry inspector who was involved in one of the first pilot programs in Atlanta stated that when she began her career forty-four years ago, inspectors "looked inside every bird, inside and outside, from every side. All they do on the pilot is they sit and watch the birds go flying by."[43] We are definitely having a hard time seeing how this is going to produce a "safer" food product. Adding to this lack of inspection, we highly doubt employees are going to be encouraged to speak up about food-safety and quality issues. According to inside sources that have filed affidavits to the GAO, the actual implementation of HIMP would be a "total nightmare."

Dozens of agencies have written to the USDA about its flawed "successful" pilot program at twenty-five plants and urged them not to proceed and expand. According to the Government Accountability Office, the results of the USDA's pilot program lack such substantial reporting that the pilot cannot be determined to be a success.[44]

Allowing the corporations to police themselves is a proven, dangerous policy. Corporations are businesses interested in making money and cutting costs. They should be required to pay and test for foodborne pathogens. Yet why would a corporation take on extraneous costs if it can get away with it without doing so and only coast through a few outbreaks here and there? Workers from slaughterhouses have come forward and stated that there are two books: one that is shown to the USDA for inspections and the other that is kept private. The two books tell very different stories about the level of sickness, contamination, and disease.

In 2002, Senator Tom Harkin tried to undo some of the damage and bolster pathogen testing to reduce risk of contamination, but his bill did not pass. Only recently in 2009 did the Food Safety Enhancement Act pass, which is considered to be the first major law addressing food safety since 1938! This law allows the FDA to take measures to prevent foodborne illness rather than just react to it as they have done for over seventy years. Prevention—what a novel idea.

Why are we not outraged like our ancestors in the early 1900s about the conditions in which our food is produced? We are allowing companies to politically influence and jeopardize our food, health, and safety. Problematically, most people do not understand what goes on behind the closed doors of the slaughterhouse and the "farms." Our food quality is jeopardized and lives are at risk, yet we are kept in the dark about how our food is produced and unaware of the industry's standards, all for a "cheap" piece of meat. According to Representative John Dingell, "A lot more people are going to have a bellyache and die" before our broken food-safety system improves.[45] America, we deserve and can do better.

Know your Sh!t Solutions:

1) *Eliminate meat from your diet or cut down on factory-farmed meat. This especially includes chicken.*

2) *Miss the meaty flavors? Try Gardein, Beyond Meat, Tofurky, or Field Roast. They taste like meat without the crap inside. You can buy these at any grocery store nationwide.*

3) *Visit these fabulous websites to jumpstart your meatless meals: www. forksoverknives.com, www.chefchloe.com, www.vegnews.com, www. vegetariantimes.com, www.ohsheglows.com, www.kblog.lunchbox-bunch.com.*

CHAPTER 6

The All-American Meal: Eating Sh!t and Drinking Pus

"Dairy products shouldn't occupy a prominent place in our diet, nor should they be the centerpiece of the national strategy to prevent osteoporosis."

~Dr. Walter Willett, Harvard University

While eating pizza and old-fashioned vanilla ice cream is considered a quintessential American tradition, eating pus is not. Yet this happens at almost every meal, as the average American eats about six hundred pounds of milk, cheese, and butter per year.[1] Americans consume more dairy products than any other food, including meat. When we realize that there is *pus* in every dairy product we eat, along with as many as 420 other chemicals, including rocket fuel, thirty-five types of hormones, and genetically modified growth hormones, dairy isn't so tasty after all. That's right, *pus*—as in the same pus that oozes from acne zits and infections, flame retardants, and about seventeen antibiotic cocktails are in our milk, butter, and cheese. We are confident that every doctor would agree that these ingredients will not make our bones big and strong. The same industrial methods and lax governmental regulations that are allowing feces to be packed with our meat are also allowing natural and added toxins from dairy cows into our milk and dairy products. It becomes not just unpalatable to think about—dairy is causing major health issues (think cancer, arthritis, and heart disease) and sucking up our tax dollars.

Got Pus?

Cow's milk is touted as an angelic superfood that we cannot live without. Dairy is not just revered for its so-called superpowers to make us healthy and strong, but also as a comfort food in the form of milk, cookies, and cheese. From a young age, we have been indoctrinated to have dairy products and milk at every meal. Every school-aged child is served a carton of milk at lunch and encouraged to drink three glasses a day. But the brightly colored containers that depict happy cows on green pastures or jumping over the moon with joy are devoid of any evidence of the industry practices used to produce milk products and the list of harmful ingredients those packages contain.[2]

What the dairy industry fails to tell us is that with every sip of milk we are swallowing *pus*. Think of that next time you pour milk over your cereal. Pus contains bacteria, white blood cells, and tissue debris. It oozes from infection sites and is one of the body's defense mechanisms against infection. Pus is extremely resilient. It cannot be boiled, steamed, or frozen out of the milk. Even though we cannot see it, *we drink it.*

The USDA and the dairy industry are well aware that there is pus in our milk and dairy products. The USDA has kindly limited the amount of pus "allowed" in each liter of milk. The USDA refers to pus in milk as the somatic cell count, or SCC, which is the measurement of white blood cells per milliliter of milk.[3] To be specific, there are about 135 million pus cells in every eight-ounce glass of milk. Let's be real here. Debating the pus limit or talking about how many millions of cells are in one glass is futile. The pus limit should be zero. Pus is gross, disgusting, and should not be allowed in our food and drink. Agreed?

The more important questions are where does all this pus come from and why is it allowed in dairy? Pus gets into our milk from cruel and unnecessary dairy practices used to produce more milk out of each cow, which results in excessive milking, unsanitary conditions, and the injection of growth hormones. Just like the meat industry, dairy has gone from pasture-based farming to housing thousands of cows in confined, crowded, factory-like conditions. In California, the leading dairy-producing state, 95 percent of dairy products come from dairy factories.[4]

Today's dairy cows spend their short lives hooked up to machines that consistently milk them throughout the day. As one can't get milk without a baby, these cows also spend the majority of their years pregnant and giving birth. Although this milk is intended for their babies, as is every mother's milk, these cows never feed their babies. Instead we drink their babies' milk. Seems a little greedy, especially since we wouldn't let any other animals steal milk from our babies.

This harsh life takes a toll on the dairy cows that now barely live to see their sixth birthdays. Dairy cows used to live to be about twenty years old. These days, dairy cows are slaughtered at around five to seven years of age, because they are crippled from calcium depletion, cannot stand due to painful foot infections, or have been so overmilked they are no longer producing the desired quantities. Since dairy cows are so exhausted and riddled with infection by the time they are slaughtered for food, they make up our lower-grade meats, such as hamburger meat. We eat these beaten-down creatures.

rBGH: Milking the Pus for All It's Worth

Today dairy cows produce about one hundred pounds of milk a day.[5] In 2012, individual dairy cows produced about 21,697 pounds of milk that year.

This is a 120 percent increase from just thirty years ago.[6] The dairy cows aren't magically producing more milk. Monsanto—the company known for its genetically modified corn and soybeans—came up with a growth-hormone stimulant called recombinant bovine growth hormone (rBGH), also referred to as recombinant bovine somatotrophine (rBST), that increases the Insulin-like growth factor, or IGF-1, in cows, so they can produce more milk. Cows injected with the growth stimulant produce up to 25 percent more milk per day. Despite studies that showed that rBGH was a public-health risk, as IGF-1 is directly associated with increased cancer, the FDA approved the use of rBGH, which is marketed under the name of Prosilac, in 1993.[7] Prosilac and rBGH is one of the main reasons there are pus, blood, and antibiotics in our milk.

While Monsanto claims that rBST is perfectly safe because BST is a hormone already found in cows, studies from the Canadian Veterinary Medical Association, the United Nations, the World Health Organization, and the European Commission's Scientific Committee on Animal Health and Animal Welfare tell a very different story. They found that rBGH increases the risk of the infection mastitis, which increases the amount of pus in milk. Monsanto's original trials of the drug also showed that their toxic effects increased lesions and mastitis. While "an increased risk of mastitis" is listed as a side effect on the Prosilac label, Monsanto continues to deny any health risks associated with its wonder drug.[8] Apparently distorting the truth can be profitable.

Mastitis is a very painful udder infection that produces liters of milk laced with pus, blood, and bacteria. About half of the dairy cows in America suffer from mastitis. Since mastitis requires antibiotic treatment, milk also contains a slew of antibiotic residues from up to twenty different antibiotics used to treat the infection. As the USDA only tests for about six antibiotic residues, more antibiotics than we care to think about are making their way onto our menus. When tested, dairy cows that became meat had residues from more than six antibiotics in their milk.

What could be hiding in your gallon of milk? Any of the following medications: "Ampicillin, Amoxicillin, Chloramphenicol, desfuroylceftiofur cysteine disulfide, Dihydrostreptomycin, Florfenicol, fluoroquinolones, Gentamicin Sulfate, Lincomycin, Neomycin, Oxytetracycline, Penicillin, pirlimycin, Spectinomycin, Tetracycline, Tilmicosin, and other compounds."[9] Penicillin is the most tested antibiotic in milk because there is a common allergy to it. How do antibiotic allergies develop? Overuse and abuse. Clearly this blatant abuse is going to limit the number of antibiotics available to us. The scary thought is every time you add a splash of milk to your coffee or eat some cheese, you have no idea how many antibiotics you are being exposed to.

The European Union, along with Canada and the United Nations, has banned the use of rBGH in cows because of the dangerous side effects. Despite industry claims that rBST is identical, it is actually at least 5 percent different from the natural hormone. This percentage, albeit small, makes a world of difference. Not only does the rBST milk contain higher IGF-1 and antibiotic-residue levels, but it also causes differences in the actual milk composition between the long- and short-chain fatty acids.[10] In fact, milk that contains the genetically modified hormones is known to go sour more quickly. This should be a clear sign that the contaminated toxins are not for human consumption. Yet to this day, the FDA has not banned its use in the United States. The FDA is aware of the harmful effects of Prosilac, both from Monsanto's own unpublished studies and from the numerous petitions the FDA has received from scientists and researchers evidencing the shoddy research backing rBGH's health claims.

Drinking Pus Makes You Sick

The United States has unwisely decided not to follow in the footsteps of other industrialized countries that have banned the growth hormone rBGH even though the negative-health implications are blatantly apparent.

According to Dr. Stephen F. Sundlof, who was a director of the FDA's Center for Veterinary Medicine back in 1999, a few years after the drug was approved, "We review all new evidence as it comes to light, and so far nothing has caused us to believe rBGH is a hazard."[11] What studies were they looking at when they came to this conclusion? Current studies, as well as those dating back to 1996, in the International Journal of Health Services found that milk from cows injected with rBGH have up to ten times the IGF-1 levels of unadulterated milk.

Why should we be worried about IGF-1? Insulin-like growth factor, or IGF-1, is a natural hormone found in both humans and cows that is responsible for stimulating cell division. Yet increased levels of IGF-1 can promote unwanted growth such as abnormal cell division leading to malignant-tumor growth, or cancer. Cows already have a higher level of these growth factors, which is a health risk. RBGH boosts these IGF-1 levels, which then passes from the cows' bodies into our milk. Higher IGF-1 levels have been shown to increase breast cancer in over nineteen studies, colon cancer in ten publications, and prostate cancer in seven publications.[12] More worrisome is that increased IGF-1 levels can block our bodies' natural defense mechanisms against fighting off early stages of cancer, known as apoptosis. Just one glass of milk a day can boost the risk of breast cancer 10 percent in adolescent girls.[13] Put simply, rBGH is a cancer-causing agent. If the FDA won't protect us from its harm, we need to protect ourselves.

We have no way of knowing whether the milk carton in our hands contains rBGH because of labeling restrictions created by Monsanto. They claim listing rBGH on labels would be discriminatory.[14] Who knew that stating a food product was healthier and didn't contain toxins was discrim-inatory? Monsanto somehow successfully sued Baskin-Robbins to prevent it from stating that its ice cream does not contain growth hormones. It even launched a marketing campaign called "Milk is Milk" to try to defend the allegations of the differences in their genetically engineered milk.[15] Unfortunately for Monsanto, its campaign can't fool us. Think health is Monsanto's concern or priority? Monsanto is making money in spite of the health risks.

The problem is that our milk products, like hamburgers, are not produced by one cow, but many cows. So the chances of having antibiotic residue, pus, and increased levels of cancer-causing growth factors in every single dairy product we eat are extremely high, if not guaranteed. To be safe, we should assume every dairy product contains disgusting ingredients that are a disaster for our health.

Milk Money from the Taxpayer

The irony of it all is that there is not a milk shortage. We would think so with the way dairy farmers continue to use the growth stimulants to manipulate cows to produce an overabundance of milk. The reality is that there is a milk *surplus* and has been for years.

Since instituting the income-support program in 2002, the government has guaranteed that it will step in and buy the remaining surplus of milk each year in order to keep dairy prices from crashing. This program keeps dairy prices high and insulated from the fluxes in actual demand. Also in 2002, the government kindly decided to use tax dollars to pay the dairy farmers funds through the Milk Income Loss Contract Program when market prices are below a certain threshold.[16] On top of the handouts dairy farmers are given, the Senate leaders decided in 2001 to introduce a plan that would give an additional $2 billion in subsidies to dairy farmers to help them through 2006. Most recently in 2009, on top of the $1 billion that had been paid in the Income Support and Price Support programs to dairy farmers, Congress decided to give away an additional $350 million of your hard-earned money to dairy farmers for handling a milk surplus. The amount of subsidies given to dairy farmers to keep them insulated from price influxes and keep them in business can cost taxpayers about $2.5 billion *each year.*[17]

To be clear, our tax dollars are being spent on buying up rBGH and pus-laden milk to keep Monsanto and dairy farmers in a business that makes us sick. This milk is sent into cold storage where it just sits there. In 2009, the government bought up $91 million dollars' worth of milk powder due to the milk surplus and declining milk sales that year.[18] Warehouses were stacked with sacks of milk powder that might not ever be used. The government gives milk that doesn't go into cold storage to the National School Lunch Program, where our children are urged to drink toxin- and antibiotic-laced milk products.

David Stockman, the budget director for former President Reagan, admitted that these dairy subsidies are "probably the single most worthless, lacking in merit program in the entire federal budget."[19] We couldn't agree more. Our dairy products should be subject to the same supply and demand as other commodities. There is absolutely zero reason or logic in promoting dairy production. To say that this is a wasteful and unhealthy cycle all in the name of scoring high prices for the corporations is an understatement.

The Dangers of Dairy

The questions we are most commonly greeted with after describing to others their milk mustaches are a sign of infection are: "Aren't dairy products good for our bones?" and "What about calcium?" Put simply, we don't need dairy for calcium or strong bones. In fact, over three hundred studies find dairy does the opposite. The shocking facts are that rather than making us healthy and strong, cow's milk can cause brittle bones and make us fat.

The science supporting dairy as healthy is junk science. The current recommendations for drinking three glasses of milk per day are not based on scientific findings. Recently the Federal Trade Commission asked the USDA, "Got Proof?" for their milk-mustache ads that prominently feature celebrities and athletes and claim that milk does the body good. Yet the USDA could not substantiate any of those claims. In fact, they found that milk does not boost athletic performance and there is zero evidence that it prevents osteoporosis and promotes strong bones. What does milk do? Filled with saturated fat, cancer-causing casein, and natural growth hormones, dairy contributes to heart disease, prostate cancer, breast cancer, ovarian cancer, type 1 diabetes, chronic constipation, sinus infections, ear infections, arthritis, allergies, osteoporosis, anemia (in children), Parkinson's disease, ulcerative colitis, Crohn's disease, multiple sclerosis, asthma, acne, eczema, and irritable bowel syndrome.[20]

Pediatricians around the world are concluding that after children are weaned from their mothers' milk, they by nature no longer need milk. Dairy is actually the leading food allergen in our children. Increasingly, studies are finding that weaning our children on cow's milk is setting them up for lifetimes of health problems. The most common childhood ailments, such as ear infections, strep throat, and attention deficit disorder (ADD), are all from feeding our children the most imperfect food. Feeding children dairy at an early age is disrupting the normal functioning of their pancreases and contributing to epidemic levels of type 1 diabetes. It seems those white mustaches aren't so glamorous after all.

Researching the funding for milk-promoting studies often reveals the National Dairy Council behind the science. Talk about a conflict of interest and unbiased resource. Unbiased studies such as a recent Harvard University study found that milk does *not* help children maintain healthy bones. "Got Milk?" does not translate to "Got Strong Bones?" In fact, the children who consumed the most dairy had the most bone fractures.[21]

All of the claims that dairy promotes healthy bones, prevents osteoporosis, and increases growth are unfounded.[22] The dairy industry and milk companies have had to retract almost all of their advertising claims, because milk is not essential to a healthy body and does not make you lose weight. In fact, 75 percent of the world's population is lactose intolerant. If dairy accomplishes none of these benefits, then it seems we need to rethink the public-health concerns that are associated with eating dairy products.

A Hearty Problem

Studies find that dairy contains the highest levels of saturated fat, or bad fat, and high levels of cholesterol that lead to heart problems. Heart disease is the number-one killer in the United States, claiming one in two people's lives. Studies show a clear link between milk consumption and heart disease.[23] Cheese is 70 percent fat, most of which is saturated fat. A little-known fact is that saturated fat causes the liver to produce more cholesterol. Clearly, eating dairy products is an unending cycle of abuse for our hearts.

Now, many people say they don't drink whole milk, just skim milk to avoid the saturated fat. Friends, skim milk is just taking the fat out and leaving the sugar and cancer-causing casein. That glass of milk just got a calorie load akin to a soda. We all know sugar plays no role in promoting athletic performance or strong bones, as sugary drinks are linked to type 2 diabetes, obesity, and heart disease.[24]

Say Hello to Clear, Radiant Skin

Hey teenagers, let's talk about that out-of-control acne. Acne affects about forty million Americans who spend about two billion dollars on treatments.[25] How many prescriptions, pills, and remedies have we all tried to get rid of those painful, red bumps that dot our beautiful faces? Dairy is a leading contributor to acne. It creates an acidic pH environment in our bodies that clogs pores and is loaded with both natural and genetically modified hormones.[26] Seriously, save your money and ditch the dairy and cheese for healthy-looking, radiant skin!

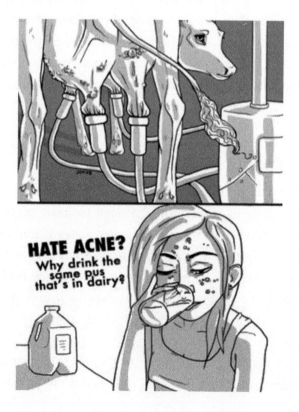

Staying Abreast of the Cure

Sadly, breast cancer is a major problem in the United States. Most people know someone who has suffered from or, in many cases, lost the battle to breast cancer. While breast cancer was previously a problem generally associated with postmenopausal women, today an increasing number of younger women are being diagnosed with breast cancer. One in eight women now has breast cancer, and only 10 percent of those cases are related to genetics. This means 90 percent of breast cancer cases are related to problems in our environment, namely our food supply. Dr. Epstein, who found that rBGH can lead to early breast development in infants and children, aptly summed up the game the FDA and Monsanto are playing with our health when he said, "The entire nation is being subjected to an experiment involving large-scale adulteration of an age old dietary staple by a poorly characterized and unlabeled biotechnology product. Disturbingly, this experiment benefits only a very small segment of the agrochemical industry while providing no matching benefits to consumers."[27]

But even in its natural, unadulterated state, dairy has growth-promoting factors that make the most hospitable environment for cancer. Fats and proteins, abundant in dairy products, cause hormonal levels to rise, which increases breast cancer risk.[28] Specifically, casein is a naturally forming animal protein in milk that Dr. T. Colin Campbell found plays a significant role in breast cancer. As casein intake increases, so does the risk of developing cancer.[29] In comparison, when patients were given soy protein, the risk of developing breast cancer decreased.

By taking the artificial growth hormones out of our milk products and, even better, removing dairy completely from our diets, we could do more for breast cancer awareness than all the pink ribbons on our food products. We need to start a new movement that actually focuses on prevention. Next time we run with our fellow mothers, sisters, and daughters for the cure, bring banners that say, "Dodge the Dairy." Others deserve to know that we possibly have the cure for 90 percent of breast cancer cases. Imagine how many mothers and daughters would be cured if we actually implemented it?

The Calcium Catastrophe

One of the more concerning myths about dairy is the claim that it promotes strong bones. Women and young girls have grown up under the illusion that if we don't drink milk or eat yogurt to get calcium, we will develop osteoporosis. Osteoporosis, or the weakening of our bones, causes 1.5 million fractures per year, of which three hundred thousand are broken hips.[30] However, there has yet to be a study that proves consuming dairy is a deterrent to osteoporosis. Reviews of over fifty studies by the American Academy of Pediatrics concluded that there was little evidence to support the claim that children need milk for strong, healthy bones. A study by the National Dairy Council found that the high protein content in dairy actually leaches calcium from our bones. This means dairy doesn't prevent osteoporosis but actually promotes it. The United States has the highest consumption of dairy products and the highest rates of osteoporosis.[31]

When Japanese women began adopting the Western diet, the rates of osteoporosis increased as their dairy intake did. In reality, the countries with the highest dairy intake have the highest rates of osteoporosis and are still obsessed with calcium intake from dairy. We are caught in a calcium paradox. Ironic, isn't it?

The truth is that dairy products are not a good source of calcium, because they are damaging to our bone health. Let us explain. We are so hyped up about getting enough calcium that we are actually getting too much and from the wrong sources.[32] There are two ways our body gets calcium—from eating calcium-rich foods (from plants, the good way!) or leaching calcium stored in the bones.[33] Our bodies like to stay in an alkaline-balanced state, but animal products produce acidic environments in our bodies. The body quickly needs to regulate and restore its preferred alkaline pH state that keeps it functioning properly. To do so, our bodies draw calcium from our bones to stabilize our inner pH balance.[34] Put simply, too much protein-rich animal foods cause our bodies to take calcium away from our bones, achieving the very thing we are aiming to prevent in the first place—brittle bones.

Friends, we are making ourselves sick by aiming to do the right thing for our health with the wrong information! Stop worrying about calcium and protein intake. As Harvard studies indicate, there are much better sources for calcium than dairy. We can get enough calcium and protein from eating leafy green foods such as kale, collard greens, and broccoli. An added benefit of these vegetables is that they are high in vitamin K, which regulates calcium.[35] Clearly, the beneficiaries of consuming animal products are the dairy and meat industries themselves and big pharma. Out with the false information that we have been fed for too long and in with the real science!

Ditch the Dairy

While hard to believe, the truth is that dairy products, with their genetic modifications, added contaminants, and their natural use of growing a calf into a full-sized cow, are linked to a whole host of health problems, including autoimmune diseases, gastrointestinal diseases, asthma, and cancers. While we have touched on the basics of the dangers of consuming dairy and how it is responsible for contributing to America's failing health, we suggest you read *The China Study* by Dr. Colin T. Campbell, *The Food Revolution* by John Robbins, *Whitewash* by Joseph Keon, and *Milk: The Deadly Poison* by Robert Cohen.

There is absolutely no benefit from eating dairy. Science doesn't support it, our health is suffering from it, and our pocketbooks are emptying because of it. Do yourself a favor and drop that dairy!

Know your Sh!t Solutions:

1) *Try holding the cheese on your pizza. Use hummus, pesto, or the many, varying, vegan-cheese flavors instead. Some of our favorite brands include Treeline, Daiya, Follow Your Heart, and Kite Hill.*

2) *There are healthier alternatives to those creamy foods we love. Avocado, a true superfood, makes an excellent creamy substitute. A sample of avocado's health benefits includes a healthy heart, sharp mind, and anti-aging and anti-inflammatory agents.*

CHAPTER 7

The United Corporation of America

"We found significant influence from the [meat and dairy] industry at every turn: in academic research, agriculture policy development, government regulation, and enforcement."

~Pew Commission on Industrial Farm Animal Production, Johns Hopkins University

Our government and its subsidiary organizations—the USDA, FDA, and EPA—are not always working in the public's favor to protect our food, but rather for the benefit of corporate interests. Agribusiness is one of the most powerful lobbies in Congress and continues to effectively "buy" favorable legislation. This is why the FDA and USDA knowingly allow feces to remain in your meat, the animals you eat to be injected with growth hormones and antibiotics, rendered animals to be put into animal feed, and rocket fuel and pus to stay in your milk—all practices that other industrialized countries such as Japan, Canada, and the United Kingdom have banned.

Although the general conception of the American public is that the FDA and USDA were created to ensure food quality for the public benefit and Congress was created to protect the public's interests, the reality is that, based on government organizations' actions, current policies work to protect the interests of the corporations in the food industry. While America was founded on the principle of freedom of speech, factory farming and agribusiness are rapidly taking away the American people's rights to free speech and safe food. Agribusiness-corporate interests are controlling America by spending corporate dollars, lobbying Congress about legislation, and silencing community voices. To restore order, it's time to stand up to USDA, Inc., FDA, Inc., and Congress, Inc. and take the money out of politics.

The USDA: Not Working for the People

President Abraham Lincoln established the USDA—the United States Department of Agriculture—in 1862. The USDA was first formed to help American farmers. While it claims it still fulfills Lincoln's vision as a "People's Department," the reality is very different, as the people's health and best interests come behind corporate interests. The USDA might touch "the lives of every American, every day," but today it does not have the positive impact that Lincoln obviously intended.[1]

On its website, the USDA claims two missions: one is "expanding markets for agricultural products" and "further developing alternative markets for agricultural products and activities" and the other mission is "enhancing food safety by taking steps to reduce the prevalence of food-borne hazards from farm to table."[2] Although on the surface these two goals aren't mutually exclusive, the USDA's activities clearly favor one over the other. Protecting our food safety has taken a backseat.

For example, let's look at the USDA's messages on cheese. On the one hand, the USDA has the consumers' best interests at heart by urging us to eat less cheese and saturated fat. It even asks consumers to consider holding the cheese on their pizza. At the same time, the USDA provides funding to the marketing group it created called Dairy Management that seeks to promote the consumption of cheese. While the USDA is asking the public to limit cheese, in 2010 the Dairy Management group partnered with Domino's to provide 40 percent more cheese on pizzas.[3] The USDA provided $5 million in funds to the Dairy Management group a year earlier. It seems the USDA is speaking out of both sides of its mouth. So which mission does it believe in, health or industry interests? Clearly, the two are not compatible. It's time the USDA picked a team.

The problems with the USDA do not stop at its mixed messaging. It has gone through massive deregulation without the public's knowledge. The Hazard Analysis and Critical Control Point Program, instituted under the Clinton Administration in 1998, is one clear example. Under HACCP, the USDA leaves regulation and inspection plans up to the food-processing plants. The USDA only checks the paper versions of the plans to ensure that the processing plant doesn't openly have any problems. After companies adopt the plans, they are presumed to be making safe food products.[4] We all know that from plan to implementation, there can be numerous problems.

This means even though the USDA never inspects the actual food products, they still receive the USDA stamp of approval. The public was never notified of this change. Like many of you, we were shocked to learn that the USDA stamp of approval doesn't actually correlate with real inspection. This means we are tricked in to believing that our food products are inspected, regulated, and safe when in fact the opposite is true.

In fact, the USDA only minimally tests food products on its own. Ann Veneman, the Agriculture Secretary appointed by President George W. Bush from January 2000 until January 2005, vetoed a program that would test all cows for mad cow disease.[5] It is important to note that Ann Veneman was linked to a company that produces the bovine-growth hormones for cows and to a major meatpacking corporation at the time she made this decision. Only twenty thousand cattle were tested in 2003 out of the thirty-five million slaughtered that year. Testing all of the animals is not impossible. Japan tests each and every one of its cows killed for human consumption to ensure a safe food supply.[6]

Aside from lax testing, the USDA has even falsified records to sell contaminated meat. Lester Friedlander, a former USDA veterinarian, spoke out and stated that he was told that if he found evidence of mad cow disease, he needed to keep that information a secret. He confirmed that the USDA has overturned laboratory tests of cows that had tested positive for mad cow disease.[7] The USDA has been known for adulterating reports and telling their employees to lie about test results to cover up mad cow disease. Secrets and lies. This is the USDA's approach to food safety.

In all fairness, conflicting corporate interests have made the USDA less powerful than we think in regulating and enforcing food recalls. During the peak of food recalls and foodborne illness sweeping the nation between 2000 and 2004, the USDA Inspector General openly admitted that the meat eaten in the United States is contaminated with sh!t and that this contamination is "continuous."[8] Where was that statement publicized? Anyone?

Despite this knowledge, zero enforcement action was taken to remedy the situation. When there were nineteen beef recalls in 2007, the USDA failed to trace the beef products back to the slaughterhouse and meat-packing processors. The USDA actually can't disclose where contaminated meat comes from, as this is considered "proprietary" information.[9, 10] In fact, if a company decides to voluntarily recall a contaminated product, they are under no obligation to notify the public. The state of Minnesota managed to trace one outbreak to Cargill. The lawsuit was settled out of court for an unknown sum, in order to prevent the public from knowing the extent of the outbreak. The twenty-five million pounds of *E. coli*-contaminated beef products recalled had the USDA stamp of approval.[11]

What is depressing is, year in and year out, food recalls and safety aren't improving. Most recently, in January of 2014, nine million pounds of beef, the equivalent of an entire year's worth of beef production, was recalled by the California company, Rancho Feeding Corp, due to lack of federal inspection that resulted in it using unhealthy animals to process meat.[12] The level of deception and adulteration, such as trimming off cancerous tumors on the animals and using fake stamps of approval, emphasizes the glaring oversight in our food-safety policies.[13]

One major problem with the ability of our governmental organizations to do their jobs is the division of labor between the FDA and the USDA that is complex and even nonsensical, which allows gaping holes for oversights. The FDA and the USDA are both tasked with the job of regulating our food system. In simple terms, the USDA is in charge of overseeing meat and poultry, and the FDA is in charge of overseeing seafood. Yet it gets quite complicated.

For instance, let's take eggs. The FDA oversees the safety of whole, shelled eggs, whereas the USDA oversees the processing of eggs and the packaging and labeling of whole eggs. The question is who is in charge when there is a safety hazard such as *salmonella* poisoning of whole eggs? It seems the USDA is in charge of regulating the facility where the eggs are produced, but the FDA is accountable for the safety hazard of the eggs themselves. Even more interesting, open-faced sandwiches are inspected by the USDA and close-faced sandwiches by the FDA.[14] Sausage is regulated by the USDA, but pepperoni is regulated by the FDA. Confused? Don't worry, we are probably just as confused as the USDA and FDA.

Although the FDA does not "regulate" food like the USDA does, the organization that is supposed to regulate harmful chemicals and substances being put into our food supply has outrageously failed. Rather than not allowing chemical substances into our food like the rest of the developed and industrialized countries' organizations, the FDA has instead decided to "regulate" the amount of chemicals allowed in our food, such as arsenic and cancer-promoting growth hormones, that have clearly been proven harmful through numerous studies.

The approach that the FDA (and USDA) chooses to take is to allow your food to be contaminated up to a determined maximum-exposure level. This does not mean that there is no hazard from ingesting these toxic chemicals or that the food you eat is free of contaminants.[15] Rather, your food is deemed "safe" by the industry's own definitions. "Safe food" is then a very relative term.

In comparison, the European Medicines Agency (EMA) that oversees food safety has a very different approach. While the USDA allows health hazards up to a level it somehow deems appropriate, the EMA only certifies use of chemicals if it is backed up by studies that prove there are zero health hazards. This is why the European countries have banned arsenic use in chicken feed. Since there is not a safe limit, the European government will not allow it to be used. In comparison, the FDA allows arsenic—a known toxin and cancer-promoting agent—in chicken feed. The tolerance level for chicken livers is up to four times as much as that for chicken breasts, thighs, and muscle tissue—the areas where arsenic is stored.[16]

The USDA and FDA are not representing the concerns of Americans. In a recent poll, two-thirds of Americans stated that they wanted more oversight of their food safety.[17] This attitude has not changed since 2007, when the same poll was issued. As recalls increasingly hit the news, more and more people realize that there is a clear problem with our current system. Despite this desire, government organizations are increasingly not complying with American interests even after the passage of the 2010 FDA Food Safety Modernization Act. Michael Taylor, the FDA Deputy Commissioner for Food and Veterinary Medicine, stated that the public's desire for better oversight will probably not become a reality any time soon. Shockingly, the issue comes down to funds and lack of resources. Mr. Taylor stated, "We will continue efforts to make the best use of the resources we have, but simply put, we cannot achieve FDA's vision of a modern food safety system and a safer food supply without a significant increase in resources."[18] We have an idea to fix the lack of resources. Let's take the billions of dollars in federal subsidies propping up the agribusiness industry and reallocate those resources to food safety. In order to achieve this solution, though, we have to get the USDA, FDA, and Congress out of the industry's back pocket.

Congress for Sale

Shocking but true: our government and legislation is heavily "bought off" by corporations. From 2005 to 2010, the ten leading agribusiness interests spent $127 million lobbying Congress and federal agencies.[19] The base of lobbyists increased to an impressive 159 people. This means there was about one lobbyist for every four members of the House and Senate. For those of us who believe in fair play and legislation that is hopefully in the best interests of consumers, we hate to disappoint you. This isn't how bills are made and passed. Although it is illegal to sell a vote, it is perfectly acceptable and legal to vote for or against a bill based on a donor's preferences. Time and again, the industry has proven that "changes in contribution determine changes in voting behavior."[20]

Let's take the Farm Bill, Federal Agriculture Reform and Risk Management (FARRM) Act of 2013, as an example to understand why our government is currently of the corporations, by the corporations, and for the corporations. The Farm Bill is the premier legislation that regulates farm policies and subsidies. This is the bread and butter of factory farming. If subsidies got cut, factory farming would fall like a house of cards.

Over the past three years, the Farm Bill has been one of the most lobbied pieces of legislation. Although 350 organizations lobbied the bill, the American Farm Bureau and Monsanto led the charge. Over the past five years, the American Farm Bureau spent $27.9 million lobbying Congress, and Monsanto spent $36 million. In total, the industries spent $57.5 million on lobbying for the 2013 Farm Bill.[21]

The American Farm Bureau Federation is the organization that claims to be the "voice of agriculture," representing the corporate interests of meat, dairy, pigs, eggs, and chickens. Yet not only does it not support family farmers, it is out of touch with much of mainstream America's interests. The Farm Bureau is notorious for blocking and opposing environmental legislation, such as the Endangered Species Act, the Clean Water Act, the Clean Air Act, the Safe Drinking Water Act, wetlands laws, pesticide regulations, and any efforts to curb global-warming emissions.[22]

Think the Farm Bureau is concerned about ensuring we have a clean and safe Earth to live on? Far from it. Rather, they are focusing solely on its corporate interests. Worryingly, the Farm Bureau has positioned itself as one of the most powerful lobbying groups in America.

Although corporations spend billions of dollars lobbying Congress, it pays off handsomely in legislation. While the FARRM Act slashed $23 billion in costs, $8 billion from food stamps, and $4 billion in cuts to conservation over the next ten years, the bill will give $7 billion in crop subsidies.[23] Crops are the main components of animal feed, which is 60 percent of the cost of factory farming. It seems the food-stamp lobby and conservation efforts didn't write big enough checks.

In politics, money obviously talks. Over the past thirty years, the number of lobbyists as well as annual spending to Congress increased from $100 million to more than $3.5 billion. In fact, each industry spends as much as $157 million lobbying Congress to support industry practices. Breaking down the numbers, for every one dollar the industry "donates" to a Congressman, the industry receives about two thousand dollars returned in subsidy payments.[24]

This could be because along with the American Farm Bureau, industry groups like the National Cattlemen's Beef Association, National Pork Producers Council, and the National Milk Producers Federation give substantial campaign donations. It is expensive to run for office, and it is well known that fundraising efforts provide ample opportunity for industry to "buy" votes. Let's take House Agriculture Committee Chairman Frank Lucas (R-Oklahoma) as an example. Among agribusiness, he is a key target and favorite. In his 2012 election-campaign cycle, he received $744,000 from agribusiness. This was almost half of his total campaign budget. Similarly, agribusiness lobbyists contributed $453,000 to prominent House Agriculture Committee member Collin Peterson (D-Minnesota) and $346,000 to Senate Agriculture Committee Chairwoman Debbie Stabenow (D-Michigan).[25] The agribusiness lobby is extremely strategic in its approach. But it's very easy to see how this campaign money can represent a substantial conflict of interest.

All of this spending means that agribusiness holds legislative power when it comes to passing or opposing legislation in its interests. This is crystal clear when we look at the proposed bills that agribusiness lobbying has had a substantial hand in defeating. For example, 2010 was a good year for agribusiness in terms of defeating environmental legislation to restore our waterways. Agribusiness—including lobbyists from Monsanto, Cargill, Land O'Lakes, and the National Turkey Federation—successfully blocked a 2010 bill that would restore the Clean Water Act's protections to all American waterways.[26] That same year, they also defeated a Chesapeake Bay restoration bill, which would have "required all polluters to contribute to restoring the ecologically imperiled health of the Chesapeake Bay, and provide billions of dollars for clean up." Naturally, agribusiness has little interest in cleaning up its messes.[27] Unfortunately, Congress also had a difficult time enacting the polluter-pay principle with corporate money in its pockets.[28] While Congress and agribusiness continue to massage each other's backs, the problem is that when it comes to the environment, we are all going to suffer the consequences. Money might fix legislation in favor of corporate interests, but we simply can't buy more clean oceans and waterways. Once they are gone, the damage is near irreversible.

In Corporations We Don't Trust: The Revolving Door

Not only does agribusiness put money into Congress members' pockets to "buy" legislation, it also infiltrates the very organizations that seek to regulate it. This notion, called the "revolving door," is where industry employees gain employment in government agencies for a short time and then often return to the industry groups. This is particularly true of the USDA. As Eric Schlosser, the author of *Fast Food Nation*, profoundly states, "You'd have a hard time finding a federal agency more completely dominated by the industry it was created to regulate."[29] It goes without saying that this creates direct conflicts of interest within the department, as the agency is notorious for employing individuals who have previously worked at the meat and dairy corporations the USDA is supposed to regulate. This revolving door has allowed the USDA and FDA to institute lax practices that result in sh!t in your meat and growth hormones and rocket fuel in your milk.

Under the most recent Bush administration, the USDA boasted a prominent staff from former meat and dairy interest groups as well as Monsanto. In fact, about a dozen of the USDA's top, high-profile officials had intimate ties to the agribusiness industry, covering the entire spectrum of interests from meat and dairy to Monsanto and large food-processing companies such as ConAgra.

Looking at the staff list, one would be hard-pressed to know it was in fact the USDA and not an agribusiness-lobbying group. For example, the highly acclaimed position of USDA Secretary was staffed by Ann Veneman, who served on the board of biotech company Calgene that was acquired by Monsanto. Ms. Veneman's Chief of Staff, Dale Moore, was the Executive Director for Legislative Affairs for the National Cattlemen's Beef Association. The NCBA is directly tied to some of the largest factory farm corporations in America, such as Tyson. The Under Secretary of the USDA, Floyd Gaibler, used to be the Executive Director of the dairy industry's National Cheese Institute. The former Senior Director and Legislative Counsel for ConAgra Foods (one of the largest food processors) was the Assistant Secretary for Congressional Relations.[30]

Monsanto, in particular, has cleverly placed quite a few of its thirty thousand employees into influential posts at government agencies.[31] If anything, Monsanto serves as a blueprint for how to infiltrate almost every high-profile position in government to serve its own interests. Consider the following:

- Clarence Thomas, a Supreme Court Justice since 1991, is a former Monsanto lawyer.
- Donald Rumsfeld, the well-known US Secretary of Defense, was CEO of GD Searle & Co, which was acquired by Monsanto.

- Margaret Miller, a FDA branch chief in the 1990s, is a former Monsanto chemical lab supervisor.
- Michael Taylor, the FDA Deputy Commissioner for policy from 1991 to 1994 and the Deputy Commissioner for Foods since 2010, is a former Monsanto lawyer and served as Monsanto's vice president for Public Policy.

Just to refresh your memory, the FDA approved the use of Monsanto's rBGH growth hormone in cows during the 1990s, despite reports of rBGH's dangerous side effects in cows and potential human-health hazards. Ms. Miller and Mr. Taylor might just have had something to do with getting that FDA approval. They also might have been influential in staving off efforts to repeal rBGH even as mounting scientific evidence from a variety of sources urged the FDA to act.

We can't judge people by their past employment necessarily, but the implemented policies that undermine the regulatory mission of the USDA and FDA in favor of maintaining high profits for corporations says otherwise. For example, the USDA continued to support the misguided EQIP programs that give conservation money to factory farms to aid in waste management. The USDA also denied and avoided testing of mad cow disease in 2003 instead of taking measures to assure the safety of America's food supply to consumers. The USDA and FDA have also continuously turned a blind eye to scientific research that has recorded the harm of genetically engineered foods and continued to support and push them onto unknowing consumers *without* labels.

Although the Obama administration pledged to help end the revolving door, it continues to staff former industry employees in extremely prominent positions. For starters, the USDA Secretary Tom Vilsack has ties to Monsanto and openly promotes genetically engineered crops. This could be one reason why, despite public support for labeling of genetically modified foods, the USDA has continuously failed to implement the provision. Staffing Michael Taylor, Monsanto's former vice president for Public Policy as the Deputy Commissioner for Foods, most likely does not bode well for

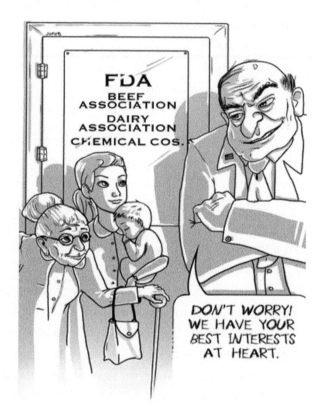

the American public. Unfortunately, this administration has failed to "close the revolving door that lets lobbyists come into government freely and lets them use their time in public service as a way to promote their own interests over the interests of the American people when they leave."[32]

Silencing American Voices

America prides itself on being a country built on freedom of speech. Corporate interests are quickly and swiftly limiting that ability. Some of the most atrocious ways they are achieving this is through ag-gag laws, which make it illegal to defame or speak out against factory-farming practices. To agribusiness's horror, undercover footage of atrocious practices in its "farms" that reveals the truth behind the factory doors made it to mainstream media.

The industry is worried about videos and photographs surfacing that show animal cruelty and filthy and barbaric conditions fit for the spread of pandemics, which could undercut its profits. Nor is it pleased that America is finding out just how disgustingly and inhumanely the animals that wind up on our plates are treated. The reason factory farms survive is because most Americans have no idea how they operate.

The agribusiness industry has responded to these revelations not by changing its practices, but by pushing for legislation that makes it illegal to showcase pictures or videos of factory farms. It has made very clear that the goal of these laws that result in jail time for offenders is to protect the industry. Now, friends, this should be a major clue that the industry is not engaging in wholesome activities. Why would it evade transparency if it has nothing to hide?

Most of us would think that these bills would never pass through and become law. How could states pass such egregious freedom-of-speech violations that work to make sure industry practices are secretive? And yet ag-gag laws passed in Iowa, Missouri, and Utah in 2011 and 2012. Ten other legislatures, including those in Arkansas, California, Indiana, Nebraska, New Hampshire, New Mexico, Pennsylvania, Tennessee, Wyoming, and Vermont all proposed bills for consideration in 2013. Pennsylvania's proposed law even criminalizes downloading photographs or videos of factory farms over the Internet.

The corporations' supposed-legal basis for these claims is the violation of their private property rights. They liken it to someone going into a person's private home with a hidden camera. That is quite a logical stretch. What agribusiness seems to be missing is that our food production is not made in private homes but in corporate practices. America, let's be honest. This has nothing to do with trespassing and everything to do with keeping the public in the dark so we know as little as possible about how food is produced. To propose this legislation in the first place is ridiculous, but to actually have it pass in certain states is preposterous. If anything, these ag-gag laws are encroaching on our civil liberties and those, rather than corporate interests, should be protected.

Silencing America's voices just begins with ag-gag laws. Agribusiness has also sought to enact cheeseburger laws, right-to-farm laws, and veggie-libel laws. Cheeseburger laws make it illegal for plaintiffs to sue corporations for obesity claims. Surprisingly, cheeseburger laws have passed in twenty-four states. The most infamous laws supporting agribusiness are probably food-defamation laws, or veggie-libel laws. Oprah Winfrey brought these laws to light in 1996, when she claimed that she would never eat a hamburger again after learning how it was produced. Subsequently, sales of beef went down, and Texas cattlemen, led by Cactus Feeders, Inc. owner Paul Engler, sued her for defamation and lost profits.[33] Apparently, the Texas cattlemen don't believe in freedom of speech. Even though Oprah won, after a very expensive and drawn-out case, the fact that a person can get sued for expressing a personal opinion based on fact goes against the very principles of America as the "land of the free, home of the brave."

And yet, veggie-libel laws have passed in thirteen states to date. If people voice that they hate Brussels sprouts or broccoli, should they be sued? Ag-gag laws seek to protect economic interests, but they are coming at an expense to American civil liberties. If we don't like the way corporations are destroying our health and our environment, and if we never want to eat chicken again, we damn well should be able to express that opinion without retribution. In case agribusiness forgot: freedom of speech is not a privilege, it's an American right.

Shockingly, the agribusiness industry has gone so far as to label those who speak out against their practices as terrorists. Dubbed the Animal and Ecological Terrorism Act, these laws provide stiff penalties for criminal conduct such as vandalism or theft when a farm is involved. While we wholeheartedly do not endorse violence or destruction of property, branding Americans as terrorists is beyond extreme. The fact that thirty-nine states have enacted eco-terrorism laws is not only mind-blowing, but also speaks to the clout of agribusiness in politics. The point of these laws is to establish a level of fear for attempting to go against these corporations that are "innocently trying to protect America's food supply." They aren't fooling anyone. Ask yourself: do these food corporations care more about their bottom lines or our health?

We can't trust an industry to protect American interests when its wallet is at stake. The industry has proven this to us time and again through pushing chemically laced and genetically engineered additives in our food onto unassuming and trusting consumers. As former US Secretary of Labor Robert Reich proclaims, "Companies are not interested in the public good. It is not their responsibility to be good."[34]

Let's be frank; the only way the food supply gets safer is when the public steps up to require corporations to disclose what is happening behind closed doors. For example, in 2009, undercover footage of downed cows, too sick to walk or stand, being forklifted to slaughter at the Westland/Hallmark Meat Company plant in Southern California led to one of the largest meat recalls in US history to date. Since downed cows can pose a substantial human-health risk, more than 143 million pounds of beef were recalled.[35] Without this footage, the industry would have continued these practices that work to endanger, not make safer or protect, our food supply.

The danger of these ag-libel laws is they undercut necessary and healthy inquiry that actually benefits consumers. All of these laws that stifle investigation and the flow of information go directly against consumer interests. America, we were born out of the fight for freedom to express our beliefs, and these very values are being corrupted by short-sighted corporate greed.

Government is supposed to protect its citizens, and yet our government has made it clear that it doesn't give a damn about our interests. The National Meat, Dairy, Pork, and Chicken Councils are taking legislative action to avoid regulation, as well as keep the public in the dark about what is in our food. Slack regulation hurts our loved ones and our planet. Don't be fooled. Do you really think our food is being inspected? It is time to enforce corporate accountability for making us and our planet sick. We are done standing by the sidelines. Let's reestablish a government of the people, by the people, and for the people.

Know your Sh!t Solutions:

1) *The chance of your meat and dairy being inspected is slim to none. Don't be fooled by labels claiming it is USDA approved. The USDA inspects plans on paper. Safeguard your family by buying organic, plant-based foods.*

2) *Don't blindly follow USDA guidelines. They are paid for by the meat, dairy, egg, and chicken councils, as well as influenced by Coca-Cola. If you trust them to give you unbiased information on what is healthy, think again. Better yet, get informed!*

3) *Do it yourself and grow your own garden. There is nothing better than homegrown veggies.*

4) *See a law you don't like? Want to protect your freedom of speech? Say something!*

CHAPTER 8

The Real Cost of "Cheap" Food

"If price spikes don't change eating habits, perhaps the combination of deforestation, pollution, climate change, starvation, heart disease and animal cruelty will gradually encourage the simple daily act of eating more plants and fewer animals."

~ The New York Times

Are we really getting the best bang for our buck when we eat meat and dairy? On walking into a grocery store, $3.50 for chicken breasts, $1.50 for a pound of ground beef, or $2.60 for a carton of eggs seems like a fantastic bargain. Not even close. When it comes to meat and dairy products, price and value are not one and the same. These grocery store "bargain" prices are deceiving, because they do not reflect the enormous, external costs to society in health and environmental costs that are not directly paid for at the cash register.

Let's take, for instance, that $1.50 for a pound of hamburger meat. To produce that meat under the factory farming system requires oil for fertilizers, abundant land to grow crops for animal feed, antibiotics to compensate for the unsanitary conditions and disease outbreaks, growth hormones to raise animals at faster rates, and waste management to truck away the billions of tons of manure generated by the animals. This doesn't include the amount of destruction left in factory farming's wake from the cost of cleaning up polluted water, the irreversible loss of biodiversity and beautiful ecosystems, air pollution, global warming, and the destruction of our natural environment as well as the staggering health-care costs to fix our bodies from eating unhealthy food.

Overall the meat and dairy industries impose the highest costs to our society among all industries across the board. Consider this: for every one dollar of animal product sold, it generates $1.70 in additional costs from environmental to health care.[1] This is nearly $7.8 billion not reflected on our grocery bills. Yet we are still paying for these in health-care costs and environmental degradation. These impacts have measurable, financial consequences. The hidden costs of meat and dairy-centered breakfasts, lunches, and dinners include $314 billion in health-care costs, $38 billion in subsidies, $37 billion in environmental costs, $21 billion in cruelty costs, and $4 billion in fishing-related costs.[2] To put the subsidies in to perspective, Big Oil only receives a meager $10 billion in subsidies.

In total, the final bill for production costs not paid for by agribusiness is at least $414 billion.[3] This price includes higher taxes, health insurance premiums, decreased value of homes near factory farms, and loss of natural resources. Next time you are at the grocery store, realize that the true price of that gallon of milk is not $3.00 but $9.00. Those pork ribs should cost us $36.00, not $12.00. Factoring in the external costs of factory farming at $1.70 per one dollar of meat, dairy, eggs, and fish sold triples the prices of the goods. We need to start paying the true "value" and cost to society of these food products.

The US Meat and Dairy industries have the sweetest business deal in history. No other industry, including big oil and tobacco, has come anywhere close to this level of governmental handouts and gotten away without paying for any of the consequences. Each time the oil industry creates a spill, it is required to foot the bill. When the tobacco industry damaged our nation's health, it had to pay Americans nearly $400 billion in health-care costs accumulated over five decades.[4] For some reason we have exempted the animal agriculture industry from the same responsibility. As a society we are footing this staggering bill for any and all of the massive problems it is creating. We think our money can be better spent on less destructive practices. It's time to realize that meat production is like the two-cent coin—it costs us more than it is worth to produce.

The High Price of the "Meat Maketh Man" Myth

Price is the most powerful determinant of how we act as consumers. The majority of us live on a budget, and so we tend to buy the cheapest food possible. Overall, the amount of money we spend on food has decreased since the 1990s. In 1990, we spent 2.4 percent of our gross incomes on food. As a society we only spend about 1.7 percent of our overall income on food today—the lowest percentage of almost every other nation. Since 1979, meat and dairy products have gotten progressively cheaper. Egg prices have decreased by 79 percent, butter by 57 percent, and bacon by 25 percent.[5] Going back to Economics 101, when price falls, demand increases. Most of the food products we buy are meat and dairy, as we presume they are the cheapest "healthy" foods.

As the prices have dropped, we have been subsequently bombarded with messages from the industry and government to continue consuming these products high in saturated fat and cholesterol. This governmental push and support for meat and dairy products above healthier food options could have a little something to do with the millions of dollars that the industry shells out to Congress.

The most frustrating realization is that our government is subsidizing all of the wrong foods for our health. Since the implementation of factory farming and the $38 billion in government subsidies to factory farms, the meat and dairy industries have been able to secure some of the lowest retail prices in history for these products. To put this in perspective, this is nearly half of the total unemployment packages paid by all fifty states in 2012. By comparison, our healthiest foods available—vegetables and fruits—do not receive anywhere near the funding that processed foods and meat and dairy products receive in both direct and indirect subsidies.

The federal government is fostering economic conditions and policies that are destroying American lives. Due to "low" meat and dairy prices, as a nation, Americans consume more meat per person, a total of two hundred pounds per year, than anyone else on the planet. We pay for it too. This ridiculously high consumption of the wrong foods is making us extremely sick and our pocketbooks poor. Obesity is a national epidemic and costs the nation $147 billion dollars annually.[6] The animal-food industry costs us $600 billion in health-care costs every two years.[7] $600 billion. Think about that number. Of the 750,000 Americans who died in 2011, one-third of the deaths were attributable to cardiovascular disease. In 2010, the bill for cardiovascular disease totaled $273 billion in direct health-care costs and an added $173 billion in indirect costs from productivity loss and premature death.[8] At our current rate of meat and dairy consumption, heart disease is only expected to increase. By 2030, experts are predicting that 116 million Americans will have their hearts broken and cost us a staggering $818 billion. What is the number-one, unanimously agreed-upon contributor to heart disease in scientific literature? Animal products.

The good news is we could save over 126,000 lives and $17 billion in health-care costs per year if we ate less meat and more veggies.[9] *Currently we are not even consuming half of the daily recommended value of fruits and vegetables.* Just increasing our daily intake of fruits and vegetables by half a cup per day could save $2.7 trillion in health-care costs. That is just half a cup! Adding everything together, the value of lives saved would exceed $11 trillion dollars. Yes, simple dietary changes really are that powerful.

The Cost of Sh!tty Food

Our current production of meat and dairy gives us not only sub-quality and unhealthy food, but also adds significant health-care costs from food-borne illness. Food not regulated by the FDA is costing us $5.7 billion and, socially, thirty thousand years of life each year.[10]

Although we tend to focus on the top heavy hitters, such as *Listeria, Campylobacter, E. coli* and *salmonella,* a research team from the University of Florida's Emerging Pathogens Institute looked at just how much the fourteen most common pathogens in our food cost us each year. Here's the breakdown by disease and cost per year:[11]

1. *Campylobacter* in poultry: $1.3 billion
2. Toxoplasma in pork: $1.2 billion
3. *Listeria* in deli meats: $1.1 billion
4. *Salmonella* in poultry: $700 million
5. *Listeria* in dairy products: $700 million
6. *Salmonella* in complex foods: $600 million
7. Norovirus in complex foods: $900 million
8. *Salmonella* in produce: $500 million
9. Toxoplasma in beef: $700 million
10. *Salmonella* in eggs: $400 million

It seems like our national stomachache is proving more expensive than we thought. Contaminated chicken and turkey products alone cost an estimated $2.5 billion and fifteen thousand years of life per year.[12] These costs don't even include the continued cost of care resulting from failed kidneys and permanently impaired immune functions. Nor do they cover the true cost of losing a family member. Let's not kid ourselves. The industry isn't responsible for any reimbursement to cover health-care costs. At minimum, they should be required to fully disclose every ingredient that goes in to our food, particularly the antibiotics, chemicals, rocket fuel, etc. Although the meat industries claim it is apparently "too expensive" to make meat that isn't contaminated, we think it is too expensive for us to eat contaminated food.

Adding to the cost of foodborne illness is the growing number of pathogens that are antibiotic resistant. Our abuse of antibiotics in livestock is costing us dearly. Back in 2000, antibiotic resistance was costing us $20 billion a year and affecting nine hundred thousand Americans.[13] Today, more than two million Americans are affected, and antibiotic resistance is costing us more than $20 billion a year in direct costs and an additional $35 billion in indirect costs from lost productivity.[14] Antibiotic resistance is killing about twenty-three thousand Americans per year despite being a completely avoidable cost. Even more frightening is this statement by Tom Frieden, the Director of the CDC, announcing in 2013 that "if we don't act now, our medicine cabinet will be empty and we won't have the antibiotics we need to save lives."[15] Imagine the health-care costs then.

The corporations will kindly tell us that jeopardizing our health is all done in the name of efficiency and profit. The net benefit of using antibiotics on animals to the producers is about twenty-five cents, which is too small to even be reflected in or impact retail sales prices.[16] We are letting the industry offload enormous costs and threaten the future of medicine over twenty-five pennies. The very near future might not have cures at the rate superbugs are becoming resistant to antibiotics. It's time to learn from history. Remember the Black Plague and influenza scares? We too are poised to let the next pandemics wipe out whole populations, thanks to antibiotics that no longer work. But not to worry because we got a bargain and only paid ninety-nine cents for that chicken sandwich. Weighing what's important to you? Agribusiness is surely not.

Marketing Money Talks

Knowing what we know about meat and dairy's health claims, it's distressing to learn that the federal government is one of the main financiers behind the marketing campaigns that push the wrong nutritional messages on the public. In fact, the government has created check-off programs that directly subsidize the marketing for meat and dairy products. The goal of these programs is to influence us to buy more animal products than we would otherwise. These check-off programs are mandatory, tax-like programs that take 1 percent of the wholesale price of food products and collect these funds to pay for research and marketing that in turn boosts animal-based product sales.[17] These funds are given to councils such as the Dairy Council and the National Cattlemen's Beef Association that then come up with the witty slogans we know so well.

"Beef, It's What's for Dinner" and "Milk: It Does a Body Good" both benefit from these check-off programs. Most Americans have absolutely no idea that these programs exist.

These check-off programs provide about $557 million in research and marketing money for animal products.[18] Although forty cents of every one hundred dollars might not seem like a lot, according to the USDA the money is well spent. The return on investment from these programs has been about $4.6 billion in sales. If we add in job creation, it brings us to a whopping $8.2 billion in return.[19] For every one dollar of check-off funds spent on advertising, it can boost sales by about eighteen dollars.

Dairy has been the biggest winner of the check-off programs, resulting in an additional $7 billion worth of milk sold. That is an extra forty-seven servings of dairy per person in the United States. The check-off program even helped the Dairy Board team up with Domino's to offer pizzas to two thousand schools. That is clearly healthy. It's not like we don't have a childhood obesity and diabetes problem. Teenagers already consume 78 percent more saturated fat than recommended. While the industry is winning from these programs, friends, we are losing. Dairy is one of the most contaminated and toxic substances that provides this industry with one of the largest bank accounts devoted just to marketing, which does not serve the public sincerely. This is just wrong. The National Dairy Promotion and Research Board boasts $389 million in check-off funds annually. No other industry comes close to having these resources. It spends $58 million a year convincing consumers that dairy is healthy.[20] Their budget is three times bigger than that of vegetable and fruit producers', which provide the delicious foods we should be eating anyway.

Although the industry is benefiting from these programs, the one at fault here is the federal government. Did you know the "Pork, the Other White Meat" slogan is actually a government-marketing campaign? That's right, the Supreme Court established in the *Johanns v. Livestock Marketing Association* case that these check-off programs and their resulting marketing campaigns are actually government speech.[21] The government decided to get involved to make the programs mandatory. In fact, every single marketing campaign is passed through the USDA for approval. While the National Pork Board might be telling us that everything is better with bacon, the overarching voice behind that slogan is our very own government.

While government and industry applaud these programs, they might want to go back and look at the numbers. Let's add in external costs and see how well these programs pay off. Since every $1.00 spent on meat, eggs, fish, poultry, and dairy generates $1.70 in external costs, that means there is an external cost of $7.8 billion not reflected in retail prices.[22] Basic mathematical comparison says that this $7.8 billion dwarfs the $4.2 billion generated in industry sales. Even including the job creation, the external costs and revenue are almost equal. The question then is, are these programs that support unhealthy practices and destroy our environment still worth it? We think not.

Survival of the Fittest

In 2011, the US government agreed to buy $40 million worth of unwanted chicken products. Apparently the demand for chicken products remained far below the number of chickens produced that year. This buyout, along with a similar purchase in 2010, gave "producers an extra $86 million in government chicken purchases above the roughly $100 million the USDA buys in scheduled chicken purchases for a year."[23] Apparently the National Chicken Council was all too thrilled with this federal bailout, stating, "At a time when the industry is under great stress due to the high cost of feed ingredients and the general economic slowdown, we appreciate USDA's willingness to step forward and acquire additional chicken." Excited? We're not smiling.

Under normal circumstances, when demand for a product declines, business has to adjust to the changing landscape and market forces. That is a basic tenet of capitalism. Instead, our government decides to prop up an industry and isolate it from market forces. Why can't we let the market regulate supply and demand like it does for other products and commodities? What is even more annoying is that the poultry industry already receives billions and billions of dollars in subsidies to pay for almost every aspect of its business. Then on top of it all, the government buys millions of dollars' worth of unwanted product and pushes this onto our children's lunch plates. It's no wonder our children's health is failing as we continue to feed them what is considered the most contaminated meat product. We are also setting our children up for failing health; chicken is high in cholesterol and saturated fat that contribute to weight problems, heart disease, and diabetes, as well as some cancers. Remember, the first ten years of a child's life directly impact his or her risk of developing a chronic disease later in life, so establishing healthy childhood eating habits is crucial.

What is a loss for our nation's children is a huge win for the chicken industry. According to the Global Development and Environment Institute at Tufts University, the chicken industry alone saved nearly $1.25 billion in feed costs from 1997 to 2005.[24] Feed is the most expensive capital cost of producing chickens. So who paid for the feed? Taxpayers. The report also found that society is currently absorbing environmental costs ranging from $2.55 to $4.00 per hundred pounds of manure for waste treatment beyond lagoon storage. If the amount of water it takes to make hamburgers was not subsidized, Americans would pay thirty-five dollars a pound instead of the enticing dollar menu they are currently paying.

Friends, this practice is the epitome of wasteful and reckless spending of government dollars. Government handouts and bailouts are an extremely contentious political issue. We argue over bailing out the banks and the auto industry, but why, when it comes to agribusiness, are we silenced and complicit in funding a clearly failing venture? Not to mention that when the auto industry received its bailout, it still had to return the money. We highly doubt the chicken industry is about to make good on its IOU.

In fact, the only reasons factory farms have survived and profited are from the expensive government handouts in the form of direct and indirect subsidies and through their ability to escape responsibility for any environmental and health problems. As taxpayers we spend a total of $38 billion each year directly subsidizing meat and dairy. By comparison, actual healthy foods such as fruits and vegetables receive a meager

$17 million.[25] Fruits and vegetables don't impose the health and environmental costs that animal products do; they reduce them.

The biggest subsidy that factory farms depend upon is the crop subsidy. The government gives subsidies to grain and soybean growers when prices fall below the price of production. "Taxpayer subsidies basically underwrite cheap grain, and that's what the factory-farming system for meat is entirely dependent on," says Gurian-Sherman, a senior scientist at the Union for Concerned Scientists.[26] It is expensive to feed animals that have been shifted from a natural diet of grass to grains. This is why it is no surprise that factory farms like to use disgusting fillers, such as crap, dead animals, contaminated food, and even newspaper for the animals' food.

How much money are we really talking about in subsidies? Consider this: taxpayers paid $161 billion in farm subsidies between 1995 and 2009.[27] But two-thirds of American farmers never saw a cent. The lion's share of these subsidies goes to factory farms. Government subsidies are skewed to promote big corporate farms rather than aid the smaller farmers who would need the most help. And let's be honest, they probably are producing healthier versions of meat and dairy products.

This "free" money results in big-time savings for the factory farms. For instance, between 1997 and 2005, the pork industry saved $947 million per year, or $8.5 billion over eight years.[28] Since grain comprises 60 percent of factory farms' capital-input costs, this subsidy makes factory farming profitable.

But wait, the government gives more. Another direct subsidy is the Environmental Quality Incentives Program (EQIP) payments to help with waste-management costs. EQIP was originally designed to help small farmers. Yet the 2002 Farm Bill opened up payments to livestock production. Big mistake. These factory farms suck up most of the EQIP payments. In a four-year time frame, one thousand factory farms received, at minimum, $35 million in EQIP funding. Today the estimated amount in EQIP funding is between $100 million and $125 million a year. To be clear, this federal subsidy that we pay for is to come up with better waste management procedures for the volumes of sh!t the animals produce.

Obviously these payments are not serving their purpose, because animal sh!t continues to seep into our water sources. Manure has damaged about one-third of our waterways. So not only are we paying for the factories to improperly manage the waste, we have to pay for the cleanup. Doesn't seem fair or even financially feasible, now does it? By subsidizing grain prices and directly subsidizing CAFOs with EQIP payments, the government is propping up an industry that costs more than it is worth.

Selling Lies

One of agribusiness's most misleading claims is that it helps stimulate rural economies. Factory farms love to claim that they create jobs. The reality is far from the truth and actually the opposite. Factory farms destroy jobs, homes, and health all in one fell swoop.

In a time when the United States wants to improve economic growth and create jobs, factory farms are not the stimulus this country needs. Economic growth in communities near hog-factory farms is actually 55 percent slower than the rest of the country. Factory farms have the highest rate of turnover due to poor working conditions. The turnover rate is 100 percent—the highest for any industry. This is after they have booted all of the local farmers out of business who are unable to compete with big industrial business. For many people, farming has been in their families for centuries. That is their livelihood. But animal factories, which clearly aren't farming, are destroying one of America's quintessential figures.

After their livelihoods are destroyed, those living in rural communities have a hard time moving away. Across the country, families are imprisoned, unable to move away from the stench of manure, because their property values have greatly declined. This comes to a $26 billion reduction in property values in total.[29] It isn't hard to understand why this happened. Who would want to move next to ten thousand smelly hogs by choice?

To add insult to injury, factory farms impose huge health costs on surrounding rural communities. The health-care cost associated with ammonia pollution is $36 billion a year. This doesn't even take into account the diminished quality of life. The stench is so bad people cannot breathe. Ammonia poisoning directly related to factory farming kills about 5,100 people per year.[30] We can all agree that factory farms would win the worst neighbor award every year.

How Much For Another Earth?

We learned at a young age that when we make messes, we clean them up. Yet factory farms are allowed to create environmental disasters and let the public foot the bill. Their messes are not cheap either. In total, from manure remediation to soil erosion, pesticides, and fertilizers, as well as climate change and property devaluation, agribusiness costs us $37.2 billion in hidden external ecological costs. Think about adding that to the price tag. That chicken, beef, and pork is actually expensive.

Let's consider the environmental price tag of the over one billion tons of animal crap from factory farming:[31]

- To clean up the soil throughout the whole of the United States from hog and dairy manure would cost taxpayers about $4.1 billion.
- Reducing water and air pollution due to manure from factory farming would annually cost about $1.6 billion. Sh!t really does smell that bad. What would happen if factory farms actually complied with the Clean Water Act? It would only cost factory farms $1.16 billion for both air and water compliance. It apparently pays less to be clean.
- How much to repair leaky manure lagoons? $2.4 billion a year.[32] In addition to the problems spilled onto us by sh!t, factory farming is severely destructive. For example, soil loss is one of our nation's more prominent environmental problems. Livestock production is responsible for 55 percent of soil erosion. While this doesn't seem like a big deal, soil erosion leads to flood damage. It also costs about $15.4 billion per year.[33] Compounding this problem is

the overuse of fertilizers and pesticides on the soil that causes runoff, which damages our waterways and creates massive dead zones in our oceans, rivers, lakes, and streams. This costs about $7.5 billion per year.

When it comes to our environment, it is hard to quantify all of the external costs. The value of nature cannot always be monetized. While we can use money to remedy some of the consequences, some of the destruction is permanent and irreversible. How can you put a price on losing an entire river or species? There are priceless losses that have a ripple effect on our environment. We are fooling ourselves if we think meat and dairy are a bargain. Clearly, the industry selling points of efficient and progressive means of producing food fall flat on their face when we look beyond the grocery store price.

Reaping Real Rewards

We don't need to be math geniuses to see that the numbers just don't add up. Meat and dairy masquerade as value meals but in reality are financial (and health) disasters. As Professor Eschel so aptly stated:

> Perhaps the best hope for change lies in consumers' becoming aware of the true costs of industrial meat production. When you look at environmental problems in the US nearly all of them have their source in food production and in particular meat production. And factory farming is 'optimal' only as long as degrading waterways is free. If dumping this stuff becomes costly—even if it simply carries a non-zero price tag—the entire structure of food production will change dramatically.[34]

What would happen if meat and dairy internalized their costs? For one, most factory farms would not survive. Their profit margins are actually so small that they would be forced to revamp their business. While agribusiness howls that this would be pushing America back about fifty years, we don't think that sounds like such a terrible alternative. Back then,

American citizens never had the chronic health problems we do today, and they ate less meat. We don't need factory farms, and we shouldn't be supporting them. Imagine how much real improvement we could make in the government if we freed up the billions of dollars supporting them?

The benefits of shifting our nation's dollars away from agribusiness and toward supporting healthy ventures are astounding and range from financial to health and environmental. For example, by reducing American consumption of meat by 44 percent, we could directly benefit from:[35]

- 172,000 fewer deaths from cancer, diabetes, and heart disease each year. Diet really is that powerful!
- $26 billion in savings to Medicare and Medicaid programs. Our taxpayer dollars are currently paying for preventable disease, friends. Let's use that money more wisely.
- 3.4 trillion pounds of reduced carbon dioxide emissions each year. We might actually be able to make a real impact on global warming. Taking shorter showers just won't cut it.
- $184 billion decline in animal food's external costs imposed on society. Yes, meat really is that expensive.

Consider this: two-thirds of our government spending on food goes toward animal-based products that the USDA and doctors around the world are saying we should eat less of. Not to mention that their production destroys our environment on a local, national, and international scale. Comparatively, our government spends less than 2 percent supporting fruits and vegetables that are known to reverse and protect against heart disease, cancer, autoimmune diseases, osteoporosis, and diabetes, to name a few.

In order to achieve significant changes, the policy of handouts to meat, dairy, and processed-junk food has got to end. Unfortunately, the passage of the 2013 Farm Bill that gives $7 billion in crop subsidies does not bode well for our future.[36] It's time the cost of the industry be reflected in the price. Just like any business, meat and dairy need to internalize their costs, change their prices, and let consumers drive demand. Maybe if we step back, we can see more clearly that the focus should not be on how to sustain our current level of destruction, but on consuming less for a better-quality product. Adding up these costs, it is clear that factory farms are not an answer to feeding the nation but a costly and, we might add, smelly burden.

Know your Sh!t Solutions:

1) *Understand that your ninety-nine-cent bucket of wings costs a lot more than it is worth. Ask yourself how much you value your health before buying the cheapest meat and dairy possible. Remember, you are so worth it!*

2) *When you grocery shop, triple the price of the meat and dairy products that are in your hand. That three-dollar gallon of milk is nine dollars, friends! That's the real price. Still want it? You are paying for it with your tax dollars.*

3) *Substitute meat and dairy with lentils, whole grains, nuts, veggies, and fruits. So delicious and less expensive. It isn't just factory-farmed meat that is unhealthy; all meat and dairy is unhealthy. Think it is too expensive to eat fruits and vegetables? Check out the book* Eating Vegan on $4.00 a Day *by Ellen Jaffe Jones to get you started.*

CHAPTER 9

This Sh!t Ain't Working

Our once-thought-of-as-healthy meat and dairy-filled meals are killing our loved ones and decimating our planet. This may be difficult to accept, but it is time to face the facts. The level of factory farming's ecological and biological destruction is now mirroring a deadly virus on the loose. We are wiping out our precious, finite resources. Put simply, this food system ain't working, not just for America's ever-expanding waistline and disappearing freshwater sources, but also for the world.

Since 2006, the United Nations and Intergovernmental Panel on Climate Change has repeatedly urged that we must curb our meat and dairy consumption by *half* in order to sustain the current levels of ecological and environmental damage that meat and dairy production causes. Have we paid attention to these warnings? No. Do most Americans know about these warnings? Probably not. But now that you know what crap is in our meat and dairy, is there a reason not to embrace cutting our consumption? Honestly, what is the worst that could happen, besides possibly creating a better world, solving world hunger, restoring our pristine, freshwater sources, preserving our forests, and creating cleaner air?

Having Tea with Africa, South America, and the Middle East

Africa, the Middle East, and South America probably seem far removed from your everyday life, but they play an integral part in every meal, snack, and drink. Our food system is a global interaction, and we can no longer afford to only consider our own neighborhood. Friends, our forests are disappearing. Our fish are being wiped from our oceans, and whether we believe in science or evolution, the facts show that our global temperatures are changing. We can guarantee that if we continue down this path, we will be fighting world wars over food and water rather than nukes and oil. The United Nations, Union of Concerned Scientists, Intergovernmental Panel on Climate Change, and World Bank have already issued warnings saying that is where our world is heading.

Let's take a visual snapshot of meat production. Every pound of hamburger meat uses up 284 gallons of gasoline, sixteen pounds of grain, about 2,500 pounds of water, and fifty-five acres of rainforest. This is what it takes to make a one pounder. One hamburger utilizes oil from the Middle East, takes grain from the starving children around the world, and destroys the beautiful Amazon rainforest in Brazil. It also impacts us here at home by using 19 percent of all fossil fuels and adding $147 billion to the health-care industry to fight obesity.[1]

We just cannot continue this type of consumption. Our resources are truly running dry. We are already consuming over 20 percent of what the Earth can ecologically sustain, and this hasn't even accounted for the UN's predicted increase in meat consumption as China and India have embarked on a path to imitate the SAD, or Standard American Diet.[2] We can try to defy this logic, but in the end Mother Nature will win. We cannot live on an Earth without a healthy, biologically diverse ecosystem. We have to immediately move away from sloppy, polluting factory farms and towards the food system of the future that is sustainable, efficient, and nutritious.

Factory Farming—The Most Unsustainable Machine on the Planet

Factory farming is not technological progress. That grilled chicken breast for dinner required vast amounts of land, torn-down forests, soybeans, fertilizers, drugs, water, and oil. But for the amount of resources going in, we are not getting an efficient output in terms of calories and nutrition. Add the additional waste and toxins emitted, and it is ridiculous that we actually call this method of producing food efficient and progressive.

In this Case, Size Matters

Factory farming is the biggest user and abuser of our land resources. What does land have to do with our meat and milk? Well, when we switched animals from eating grass like they were born to do to eating grain, we needed land to grow the crops. According to the UN, one-third of the total arable land in the world is used to grow crops, such as soybeans, grains, and corn for animal feed.[3] Just imagine, a quarter of the Earth's land is dedicated to feeding the animals we eat! The total amount of land used to grow feed crops and graze equals about twelve million square miles, or the size of the whole continent of Africa.[4]

There are a few teeny, tiny issues with dedicating land the size of Africa to growing crops for animals that we eat. The first problem is we are over-using the land and inundating it with so many chemicals from fertilizers to pesticides and insecticides that we are destroying the natural qualities of the soil that keeps the land healthy and able to produce crops. This over-exhausting soybean and grain production and extensive grazing cause soil erosion and desertification. Our soil is turning to crap!

Livestock is responsible for half of all soil erosion. The United Nations found that seventy-five billion tons of soil is lost in the United States per year, which costs about $400 million dollars per year. What is the big deal with eroded soil? When the soil becomes eroded from overuse, it can no longer grow crops. Forest soil, in particular, is already nutrient poor. This means soil from these sources only lasts a few years before farmers have to move on to new land, which results in more land having to be cleared to produce more crops, and the endless cycle continues. The constant cycle of degradation of the land and then the need for additional land is a driving force behind a massive second problem: global deforestation. *We have to cut the crap, not the trees!*

The poster child for deforestation is the Amazon Rainforest. Half of the Amazon, along with its valuable medicines and rich biodiversity, will be gone forever by 2030 if we continue at our current rate of obliteration. The speed at which we are clearing the Amazon is so rapid—6 million acres annually—that NASA photos from space can visibly show the demolition.[5] The Amazon, however, is not the only area being destroyed by Brazil's ever-growing meat production. Brazil's *Cerrado* is almost completely gone. Eighty percent, or four million acres, of the once rich, biologically-diverse forest is now being used as cattle pastures and land to grow feed crops.[6] Brazil is rapidly becoming the largest producer of meat products, and the United States is the leading importer of beef from Brazil. See how our meals have a global significance?

While the Amazon and Brazil are the faces of deforestation, this destruction is happening worldwide, as other countries race to imitate America's awful example of food production. China is on the fast track to turning its country into a toxic desert. As China ups its livestock production, it is clearing away land for feed crops and grazing at an astonishing rate. Each year, land equivalent in size to the state of Rhode Island is being cleared to produce meat. With the land go the exotic, unique, and breathtaking animals that call these forests and habitats home.

We are facing the sixth-largest mass extinction in history as ten thousand species disappear each year due to factory farms. This is pandemic, virus-level annihilation. Deforestation and land-use changes from factory farming are causing up to five hundred times greater than normal extinction rates than in the past. The impact of losing our forests does not just affect the immediate animals in the vicinity.

Deforestation impacts fish in our oceans. Trees do more than just release oxygen that we need to breathe. They help mitigate climate change by absorbing carbon dioxide. When the trees are no longer around to absorb the carbon, the carbon either sinks into the ocean or is released into the air, contributing to the increase in carbon dioxide in our air. When the carbon sinks into the ocean, it changes the pH balance of the water, making the ocean more acidic. Our fish are dying because they cannot live in an acidic environment. Increased acid in our oceans bleaches the absolutely stunning barrier reefs, destroying the homes of millions of ocean creatures.

What is the big deal with losing some bugs, fish, and exotic animals you have probably never seen before? Remember basic science in school where we learned about the food chain? When you wipe out massive sections of that, it creates a ripple effect that throws off the entire balance of the global ecosystem. Every living creature is affected by every single bug, insect, frog, bird, and fish that disappears from our Earth. We are completely restructuring the entire ecological system, and the consequences are dire.

The Real Hunger Games

We have about seven billion people in the world and grow enough food to feed nine billion. Yet there are about 925 million people, or one in seven people, who are starving worldwide. There is something terribly wrong with these numbers.[7] While hunger and starvation are complex, global issues, factory farming creates a major problem with distribution of our food sources. Think about this: if we reduced meat consumption by just 10 percent, a miniscule amount, we could feed one hundred million more people. Putting an end to hunger worldwide is a realistic goal, and it starts with taking our food back from the animals that are devouring the majority of our raw-food sources.

It makes absolutely zero sense that we feed 80 percent of all the grains and soybeans grown in the United States to cows, chickens, and pigs that become food. Worldwide, the meat and dairy industry uses 97 percent of all soybeans produced![8] We are only getting 3 percent of the grains and soybeans available. Since we do not grow enough grain and soybeans in the United States to feed all of our animals, we import a large portion of it from developing nations. Instead of feeding their local communities, they are shipping the grain to the United States for our buckets of chicken wings. Call us greedy, but somehow this allocation of food seems a little unfair. The irony is that when we eat meat, we are only getting 10 percent of the calories the animal consumed. This means 90 percent of what these animals eat comes out as waste![9]

Agribusiness will argue and say factory farming is the way to feed the world. By producing more meat and dairy products in as short a time and as cheaply as possible, we can feed more people and make food more affordable. Sadly, this logic falls extremely short of the truth. Every two seconds a child dies from hunger.[10] There are about sixty million Americans without enough food, and the number is growing, not to mention that meat and dairy are the least nutritious foods to feed our world.

Factory farming depends upon growing and slaughtering as many animals in as little time as possible to make a profit. To achieve this laser-fast turnover, the animals require a tremendous amount of food in order to get fat and ready for slaughter as quickly as possible. Instead of relying upon the animals' natural, grass-fed diet, factory farms feed animals fattening grains and agents that nature never intended for them to eat and are very hard for their stomachs to digest. We are using up massive amounts of resources, getting fewer calories per input than if we directly ate the grains, *and* we are eating less nutritious products. This is a lose-lose situation.

If all the grain and soybeans that are produced for livestock were given to humans, it would feed 1,400,000 people in the United States.[11] A United Nations report, *The Environmental Food Crisis*, estimated that if current meat production per capita was reduced in the industrialized world and restrained worldwide to the year 2000's levels by 2050, we would free up enough tons of cereal to feed *one billion* people in 2050.[12] If we changed the land used raising beef to growing vegetables, we could feed twenty-two times the number of people.[13] Clearly, we have the food resources to solve our hunger games. As the population has topped seven billion with indications of only increasing, we must reevaluate how we are using our existing food resources.

Water Wars

The world is in a water crisis. Countries are already fighting over access to clean water. While we assume water is a replenishing and abundant resource, clean, *fresh* water is scarce. Ninety-seven percent of our planet is water, but only 3 percent is freshwater. Of this 3 percent, less than 1 percent can be used as drinking water.[14] Not only are the animals hogging all the food sources, they are using and contaminating our freshwater sources. Globally, livestock uses 8 percent more water than humans. Considering animals' high consumption of water and resources, as seen in the Ogallala Aquifer, which is now half depleted, it is fast becoming a bleak situation. We are heading toward water wars in the very near future.

Nearly half of all the water used in the United States goes toward raising animals for food. The animals destined for your plate consume about 2.3 billion gallons of water per day, or about eight hundred billion gallons per year.[15] While these are big numbers, they do not include the rivers, streams, and aquifers that factory farms frequently contaminate with animal feces. Those numbers just account for all of the water usage it takes to get that steak on your plate: from watering the crops that are used to feed the animals to watering the animals. Of the fifty-six million acres of land that farmers irrigate for crops, twenty-three million of those acres are used for livestock feed. It takes about twenty-eight *trillion* gallons of water to irrigate those acres every year.

Let's make an easy comparison. It takes about 2,500 gallons of water, depending on the country, to make one pound of hamburger meat. It only takes twenty-five gallons of water to produce one pound of wheat. The math is not hard here. It takes about one hundred times more water to produce meat than healthy, nutritious grains. Needless to say, this substantial difference is problematic when millions of people are already living in water-stressed areas.

As the population is expected to reach nine billion by 2050, our water supply will become an ever-more precious and scarce resource.[16] Currently 1.1 billion people in the world do not have access to clean water, and another 2.5 billion do not have access to proper sanitation. In the United States, we recently had one of the worst droughts in history. Our grass shriveled to dark brown. Our crops died. Food prices spiked. Quite a foreboding preview of the future that we would like to avoid. There is a logical answer here to prevent water wars from happening.

Fuel in Our Food

While America, and largely the rest of the world, focuses on gas-guzzling SUVs, we are overlooking some of the biggest culprits of oil consumption: the cows, chickens, pigs, and lambs. A grain-fed beef steer will require 284 gallons of oil in its short fourteen-month lifetime before being slaughtered.[17] It takes eleven times more fuel to make one calorie of animal protein than one calorie of plant protein. With gas prices today eating into our paychecks, we would never dump gallons of gasoline on the floor for sport. But that is what we are doing when we eat meat and dairy products.

Our meat and dairy factory farm system is literally fueled by oil. We are not just talking about transportation and trucking food products to our grocery stores. When grain replaced grass, farmers turned to twentieth-century industrial technologies such as synthetic fertilizers, toxic pesticides and herbicides, and hybrid and genetically modified crop varieties to boost harvests.[18] This use of corn and grain as animal feed requires the heavy use of chemical fertilizers. Chemical fertilizers are made from oil.[19] By switching food animals away from their natural, grass diet to grains, we essentially switched livestock from solar-powered beings to grain-fed, fossil-fueled machines. All of this toxic crap gets into your cells when you eat meat and dairy.

Today, meat and dairy production uses 19 percent of the fossil fuels in the United States. About half of the energy used to create the glorified American hamburger comes from the production of the feed. Thirty-three percent of our land is maintained with fertilizers. In itself, fertilizer production is energy intensive, as it takes energy to bind the nitrogen-gas particles in the atmosphere. A sad incongruence is that with the amount of energy used to create fertilizers, about half of the fertilizer is lost through volatilization, leaching, and runoff from oversaturation.[20] These runoffs are killing billions of fish and contaminating our water supplies. As the United States imports the majority of its fertilizers, fertilizer incurs a huge transportation cost.[21] The scale of this problem is massive.

Adding insult to injury, using massive amounts of fertilizer not only consumes oil, but also produces harmful gases that pollute our air. One study found that "fertilizer production for feed crops alone contributes some 41 million tons of carbon dioxide (CO_2) annually—the equivalent of that produced by nearly 7 million cars."[22] This is why researchers Gidon Eschel and Pamela Martin at the University of Chicago found that a meat-eater who drives a Prius uses more fossil fuels than a vegan who drives a gas-guzzling SUV. Looks like it's time to "green" your diet, *not your car.*

Ironically, factory farming's reliance on fossil fuels goes against the very tenets of its foundation to create a more independent America. Aside from placing America's food security in a vulnerable position by relying on other countries, such as the Middle East and South America, our world's natural reserves of fossil fuels are drying up. We simply cannot continue guzzling oil for our food indefinitely.

Factory Farming Stinks

Global climate change has the potential to kill 150,000 Americans over the next decade. Air pollution from climate change will become a "bigger global killer than dirty water," killing an estimated 3.6 million people a year by 2050, according to the most recent Organization for Economic Cooperation and Development (OECD) report. Climate change is one of the most significant environmental issues of our time, and our meat and dairy diets contribute more to our changing climate than all transportation worldwide. In fact, you can drive to the moon and back 114,000 times, and you still will have released less carbon dioxide gases than the US factory-farmed chicken industry releases annually![23]

We need to make it clear that climate change is *not* all about carbon dioxide. In fact, it is the least dangerous of the greenhouse gases. Methane is twenty-five times more potent than carbon dioxide and remains in the air anywhere between nine to fifteen years.[24] Nitrous oxides have three hundred times the potential of carbon dioxide to warm the Earth.[25] What produces methane, ammonia, and nitrous oxides? Factory farming!

The majority of factory farming's most-potent greenhouse-gas emissions—i.e. ammonia and methane—come from the billion tons of animal manure and flatulence or, bluntly, cow farts. Thousands of open-air cesspools dotting the American landscape release toxic methane gases that add to climate change. The more than 160 gases released by these lagoons are so toxic that an entire Michigan family drowned in a pig-sh!t lagoon trying to save each other from the toxic fumes. Talk about a crappy way to go.

It seems silly, crude, and downright crazy to say cow farts add to climate change, but it is the truth! Grains make cows super gassy. Instead of logically dealing with this problem, a company is developing a gas pill for cows to take with their meals. Some researchers are also genetically modifying cows in their laboratory to design one that can handle all that gas. But let's be real, do we really need to go that far to cut the gas? There are obviously smarter and less ridiculous solutions.

Worldwide, cows produce about eighty-six million tons of methane a year.[26] Since cows make up 30 percent of meat consumption in the United States, and the average American consumes six hundred pounds of dairy per year, the amount of methane released from cows passing gas is significant enough to add substantially to climate change. In fact, methane released from cows is so powerful that in Germany, gassy cows caused a methane buildup so high it caused the warehouse to explode. Who would have thought that possible?[27]

Meat consumption had tripled between 1971 and 2010 to about six hundred billion pounds and is expected to double by 2050 to about 1.2 trillion pounds of meat per year. We are already experiencing a significant change in weather patterns. The polar vortex of 2014 and heat wave of 2013 are just the beginning. These massive switches will place even more pressure on our food, water, and land resources.[28]

So, what can you do to help reduce the threat of climate change? Studies by the Environmental Working Group show that eating one less burger a week is the equivalent of taking your car off the road for 320 miles.[29] That is just one burger a week. If a four-person family skipped their steak dinner one day a week, it would be as if they didn't drive for about three months. You really can make that big of a difference! While these statistics focus on meat, the answer is *not* to eat more dairy. Dairy comes from cow's milk. Milk protein and fat were only designed for newborn babies anyway. Creating a better world can start with yummy soy, almond, or coconut milk at breakfast.

The Cycle of Crap Must End

Worldwide, the livestock sector produces 586 million tons of milk and 285 million tons of meat.[30] Factory farming and the livestock sector arguably have the largest human-induced destructive impact on our planet.

We are losing species, killing our oceans, degrading our land, tearing down our forests, polluting the water, sacrificing finite resources, and changing the entire climate just so we can have sausages and eggs for breakfast and cheeseburgers at lunch. Somehow this does not seem to be a good trade-off. What we eat directly determines how long our resources will last, the quality of the water systems, the number of hungry people, and the overall state of our environmental and public health systems. At this moment, the future awaiting us is not looking too bright with higher health costs, more antibiotic-resistant bacteria, animal-factory virus mutations, eroded farm land, dirty water, and a degraded land robbed of its nutrients. We have the recipe for a food system that will keep us happy and healthy and our environment pristine and green.

Know your Sh!t Solutions:

1) *Cut down on your meat and dairy consumption. Forgoing one burger or chicken dinner a week will impact the environment and make your heart healthier. Even better, eliminate meat and dairy altogether. Read* Rethink Food: 100+ Doctors Can't Be Wrong *and have more than one hundred doctors explain why a vegan diet is the very best for your health!*

2) *Think globally! What you eat for breakfast, lunch, and dinner affects our water, air, land, and hunger worldwide.*

3) *Give a healthy vegan meal to a hungry person in need. Check out our resources for more information and delicious plant-based recipes!*

CHAPTER 10

Cut the Crap; Change the World

"We as a society are on the edge of a great precipice—we can either fall to sickness, poverty and degradation, or we can embrace health, longevity and bounty. All it takes is the courage to change."

~ Dr. T. Colin Campbell, The China Study

It's time we take a good, hard look at our society. What have we become? We are inflicting unwarranted cruelty on voiceless, beautiful creatures, abusing our technological advances in medicine, unheeding warning labels, protecting the use of toxins and carcinogens in our food, deceiving ourselves on food safety and health, abusing our finite resources, and ravaging our environment. All of this in the name of profit from meat and dairy. Ask yourself: is it really worth it? We don't think so. Our society is far from the ideals and virtues of a progressive, democratic, and capitalistic country that we so pride ourselves on being. This is the real America we are living in, and the home next generations are inheriting.

This information is not new. Many great minds before us have written about the horrors of factory farming and the problems with our food system. Yet it takes more than just science and facts to create a change. It takes action and leadership. These issues are not at the forefront of America's young minds and are often corrupted by industry propaganda. For burgeoning young leaders, we need to change our food system for the better. We cannot afford to tip the scales further in favor of evolutionary disaster. The courage to change and demand better food and transparency begins with each one of us. We do not have to accept what is handed to us by companies. Each one of our actions, whether big or small, can have a tremendous ripple effect to create much-needed, positive change. It's time to show the food corporations that we mean business by using the power of *not* buying their products.

Luckily, the pressing food, health, and environmental problems facing us today are interconnected and therefore have a combined solution. Who doesn't love simple solutions? As we have said, never before have we consumed such high volumes of meat and dairy, and we have never been such an unhealthy and disease-ridden society. As our consumption of meat and dairy increases, so have our environmental problems. This is not a coincidence. At the beginning of the twentieth century, Americans ate 120 pounds of meat per year. Now we are eating nearly double that amount.[1] Our dairy consumption has quadrupled! It all comes down to rethinking how we eat and cutting through propaganda to realize the truth about our food. We have the power to change not only our own lives, but also industry practices that are wreaking havoc on our health and homes. Already we are implementing the positive changes of renewable energy, recycling, and new technologies. Making dietary and lifestyle changes is the same as changing a lightbulb. It really is that easy.

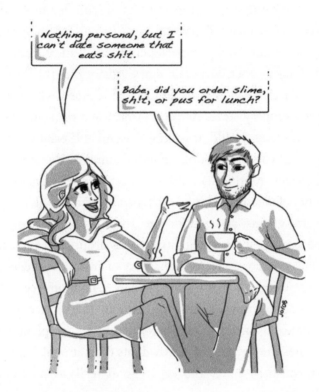

Life Is About Tasting the Rainbow

The key to a healthier you is healthier food. We understand that learning about our health and food-safety problems can feel overwhelming and, quite frankly, mind-blowing. We also had the experience of sitting back and thinking, "Great, now what?!" Most of us have no idea where to start, how to shop, or what to eat. But friends, don't despair! We have been in your exact position, and we know how easy it is to make simple, daily changes.

For some, this is a big step and completely life altering. But isn't that the point? We want a healthier, happier life, which means dropping the food that just doesn't make the cut. Do yourself (and the animals) a favor by saying goodbye to feces-filled meat, chemical-laced processed foods, and pus-filled dairy products. So now what do we indulge in? The entire rainbow is at our fingertips! From veggies to fruit, legumes, grains, and nuts (as well as soy-based dairy and meat products), the opportunities are endless. We should be experiencing the tastiest (and healthiest flavors) food has to offer. Meat and dairy are not them.

A great place to begin is to familiarize yourself with the vegetable section at the grocery store. As most Americans eat significantly fewer vegetables than they should, it will be a useful and exciting new experience for many of you. Don't be afraid to try something new. Kale might be one of the newest (and best) fads, but it really does have an enormous amount of benefits to offer. Love kale? Also try chard, bok choy, mustard greens, collard greens, and cauliflower. These cruciferous vegetables are some of the healthiest, cancer-fighting foods around. Try to eat as many different colors as possible. All the colors of fruits and vegetables offer different phytonutrients that restore our DNA, fight off free radicals, and bolster our bodies' immune systems. One of the most comprehensive studies to date on antioxidants in food found that plant foods have sixty-four times the number of antioxidants than animal-based foods do, including meat, fish, dairy, and eggs.[2] Food really is medicine for the mind, body, and soul.

A common misconception is that vegetables are boring. Yet they are some of the tastiest foods around. Giving up meat and dairy does not mean living on salads either; we just don't realize it, because we don't focus on cooking vegetables. It's not complicated. Just like you used to marinate meat to eat it, you can dress up vegetables with an array of herbs and spices that bring out their delicious taste. The best part? Most herbs and spices are an amazing source of antioxidants and phytochemicals that promote health at every meal. For instance, some of our favorite spices, such as cinnamon, can help keep sugar in check for diabetics, and turmeric, a key ingredient in curry, is a powerful anti-inflammatory agent that works to keep cancer at bay. Additionally alliums, such as onions and garlic, are powerful and potent defenses against inflammation and cardiovascular disease. While garlic cloves are great for the heart, we don't recommend eating them right before a date, especially a first date! First impressions are everything and eating a whole-food, plant-based diet will make you irresistible, radiating health inside and out. (Be sure to try our recipes at the end to get you started.)

If cutting meat out cold turkey is a bit challenging, then try participating in Meatless Mondays or reduce your meat and dairy intake by 50 percent. There are amazing meat substitutes such as Beyond Meat, Gardein, and Tofurky that can help during the transition period. While we don't endorse eating meat because we have your best interests at heart, if you do buy meat, know where it comes from and don't support factory farms. Don't be fooled by labels. It might not say "Tyson," but you have to remember that big agribusiness players like Tyson own smaller companies that appear to be local. If you are not sure if something is grass fed and organic, ask! If your store does not sell organic or locally raised meat and dairy, ask for it. Stores will gladly provide what consumers want to buy, so make a point of speaking up for humanely raised foods and fresh, local products. Again, we have to stress that just because it says cage free does not ensure that the hens did not receive drugs throughout their lives or weren't bred in crowded conditions. A good indication is to look for the Humane Farm Animal Care label.

If we were to pick one animal product for you to ditch first, it would be dairy. Dairy is one of the most contaminated foods that masquerades as healthy. We understand how hard this can be to eliminate. Dairy is naturally addictive. It actually contains casomorphin, which acts in a similar way to heroin or morphine in our bodies.[3] But just as we know heroine and morphine aren't good for us, our dairy product habit needs to be kicked.

Dairy products are everywhere, and it can be so frustrating how milk fat is snuck into so many of our foods. Even foods we least expect, such as crackers, bread, and salad dressings are tainted with the dairy disaster. Have hope! You can choose delicious, nondairy and soy-product versions over dairy products. There are thousands of recipes for delicious snacks, desserts, and meals that are made without all the crap and are just as creamy. You won't even know the dairy is missing. If you don't have time to cook, you can order online or go to your local grocery store to pick up these yummy treats and meals. If nondairy is something to work toward, choose local and organic dairy. This will give you the best chance of limiting the amount of pus you drink, since local and organic dairy cows are not given growth hormones that promote infection.

Old habits die hard, so changing how we eat is a gradual process. Don't get frustrated or give up in the beginning. Take baby steps, and on the way you will experience how great you feel when you begin to cut out the crap. Choosing to cut out meat and buy more veggies, grains, legumes, and fruit or choosing to only eat organic meat, as well as choosing nondairy products will show the meat and dairy industries that enough is simply enough. Get shopping, make dinner, and have some friends over to enjoy your feces- and pus-*free* dinner and dessert! We promise you won't look back.

Cheap Is Expensive

For many of us young professionals or college students, living on a budget means eating the cheapest food possible. Doesn't it seem ironic that we tend to invest so much time and money into our careers and education but very little into our own bodies? It's time to learn to invest in our health. It's very easy to take good health for granted, because we will only experience the repercussions or healthy success years down the line. Yet, just as it takes time to be at the top of our game, our bodies need us to take the time to fuel them properly. We will never be the best if we are operating on sub-optimal fuel. Subsidies have made it so the cheapest food available is also the unhealthiest. The newest research shows that eating healthy costs $1.50 more per day, or $550 per person over the course of a year.[4] In the long run, this could be financially prohibitive for some people, especially those with families. At the same time, let's think about how many three-dollar Starbucks coffees we drink each week. That's two days of eating healthy. Eating healthy does not have to be expensive. It is actually possible to eat a plant-based diet on four dollars a day. Beans, rice, legumes, and bulk vegetables are nutritious staples. More importantly, this disparity evidences just how important it is that we vote with our dollars so the food that is good for us is more affordable.

In college? There is never a better time to start changing your diet. You will need to be on your A game to get the grade. College students are known for following the CCC diet of carbs, caffeine, and candy. However, after learning about the harmful effects of meat on our health and environment, one in five college students have ditched meat from their dinner plates and are holding the cheese on their pizzas.[5] Most colleges these days cater to vegetarians and vegans. If your campus is still living in the past, join the Real Food Challenge. The Real Food Challenge seeks to take the junk off our college campuses and put grains, fruits, and veggies back onto the plates.[6] Now on three hundred campuses across the country and growing, the Real Food Challenge shows that young people have a voice that can change food options on campus. College is the best time to explore food options, and you have the most amazing networks and resources at your fingertips. Not to mention, college students hold $300 billion in spending power. Collectively, you are more powerful than you think.[7] Use it.

Fast Food No More

We know the feeling of driving down the road with your stomach growling and seeing those golden arches in the distance. Your stomach lurches, and oh what you would do for some French fries or a burger right now. Stay on the road! The fast-food industry is not only extremely unhealthy, but it is also a major supporter and driving force of factory farms.

For those young professionals and parents who have spent an entire day working and just want to reach for the nearest fast-food offering, we've been there, done that. Be honest with yourself. Have you ever felt great after eating those greasy nuggets that somewhat resembled chicken? It's not worth it.

Since fast-food chains are the main buyers of animal products from factory farms, by choosing to pass up the drive-through you are saying no to crappy food and the crappy-food system it perpetuates. A recent Yale study found that less than 1 percent of children's meals at fast-food restaurants could qualify as healthy.[8] Our children deserve so much better, especially as food is critical to development. That ninety-nine-cent dollar menu is a ruse, as you now know that your "cheap" food comes at an untold global, environmental, and health price.

Cut the desire for greasy fast food and throw your own (veggie) sandwich together at home for lunch. It is cheaper, healthier, and won't leave your car or you smelling like a fast-food dump. Also try cooking big, delicious meals such as veggie lasagna, stew, stir-fry, and soup on Sunday. Then during the week, after a long day all you have to do is thaw, heat, and serve. Not sure what to make? Look at our recipes and resources page.

Down with Pus, Down with Feces!

For those of you who like a more active approach and are burning with the knowledge to make profound impacts on this agribusiness industry, start making the protest signs for the Hill. Along with voting with our forks, we must change the laws and enforcement procedures to ensure our food safety. Unfortunately, unless corporations are forced to amend their ways due to legislative action or public outcry, rarely will any voluntary, positive action take place. This starts with us banding together and bombarding our congressmen and women with the changes we want to see.

We have compiled a list of changes that esteemed bodies such as the Pew Commission, World Health Organization, and the UN have suggested.[9] These changes are:

- Phasing out the use of antibiotics and other additives, such as slaughterhouse waste, blood, and manure fed to animals
- Phasing out the use of growth hormones for dairy cows and pigs
- Phasing out manure lagoons as waste storage and forcing more efficient and environmentally friendly storage facilities
- Regulating pollution and spills from manure lagoons and factory farms

- Increasing the USDA and FDA staffs to regulate the dairy and meat industries
- Fining and closing all CAFOs that violate animal rights or food-safety measures
- Ending air emissions programs that allow factory farms to violate air-quality standards
- Allowing governmental regulations of factory farms through zoning laws
- Ending veggie-libel laws
- Increasing competition and enforcing antitrust and anticompetitive laws to disperse the concentration of corporate power in the livestock and dairy markets
- Supporting those facilities that practice animal welfare and animal rights
- Ending the farm subsidies under EQIP to factory farms, which currently hide the true cost of producing food
- Enforcing environmental laws through the Clean Water and Clean Air Acts that make the corporations liable for damage to the environment and subject to stricter punishments for violations
- Reducing the level of feces allowed in meat
- Holding processing plants liable for any meat found containing *E. coli*, *salmonella*, etc. and requiring the slaughterhouse and factory-farm companies to step forward and claim responsibility for that meat, as well as an accurate account of where it was shipped
- Holding the actual corporation, rather than the farmer, liable for all environmental and health damage that is connected to its facility

While it might seem like campaigns and letters to Congress go nowhere, think again. Local and national groups challenging the laws are having success! Jerry Nivens and a few supporters successfully pushed New Mexico to enact the most progressive dairy-water regulations laws to date. It all started with a petition.

When your Congressman or woman receives letter after letter and campaign notice after campaign notice asking for healthier food and better regulation of agribusiness, he or she will begin to take notice and maybe even act with vigilance on your behalf. Congress and state legislatures will eventually have to get out of bed with agribusiness leaders and respond to the actions the public is alarmed by.

Without these legislative changes, the agribusiness corporations will continue to pollute our air, soil, and waterways with the animal crap that makes us sick. We cannot afford to waste time. Organize a group in your local community to start protesting this injustice that is levied on each one of us, and demand to know how your food is raised in animal factories.

Ensuring Americans Know Their Sh!t

Poll after poll cites that most Americans have absolutely no clue about where their food comes from, how it is produced, or what's in it. This lack of knowledge is what factory farms and agribusiness thrive upon, because they understand if the public knew the full truth there would be outrage. Look what happened when we found out about the "lean" beef trimmings or what has come to be known as pink slime in 2012. When Americans learned that this filler wasn't 100 percent beef and was sprayed with ammonia to kill off the *E. coli* and other harmful pathogens, there was such a strong backlash that it forced the USDA to allow schools to only serve it by choice. Guess what? Schools, fast-food companies, and grocery-store chains opted out of pink slime because of the public outcry.

Education and awareness are some of the most effective tools to create a better food system. There are so many resources that you can use to educate yourself and others about what is happening. Technology has made it infinitely easier to share information these days and spread awareness in a second. Please look at our resources pages that details organizations helping to change our broken food system and the books and reports that taught us our sh!t.

A Better World Begins with Breakfast

Ever dreamed of making a positive change in the world? You can do it every day, three times a day. It is our decision whether we preserve America the Beautiful or let it disintegrate into a pile of crap. As we approach a new age of climate change and water and food scarcity, the future health of our planet and the health of America's citizens rests in the hands of individuals taking action to change how their dairy and meat are produced and calling on agribusiness leaders and government to take the feces out of our meat, freshwater sources, ecosystems, land, and air. It is time to take back control and choose action over apathy, voices over silence, and compassion over cruelty. By speaking up, we will show the public officials that we know our sh!t, and we want better for us and our planet. Together we can implement the food system of the future!

Know your Sh!t Solutions:

1) *Try one of our delicious, plant-powered recipes. From pancakes to Thai curry to All-American, decadent, chocolate cake, when it comes to starting your plant-powered journey, we've got you covered.*

2) *Vote with your dollar at the grocery store for humane choices. Every item you place into your grocery cart does and can have a ripple effect. Let's vote for healthy, clean food!*

3) *Eliminate fast food from your diet—it's gross anyway.*

4) *Cook a plant-powered meal at least once a week, and share it with family and friends.*

The Meaty Truth Recipes

There are so many delicious foods that we can eat when we ditch the meat and dairy crap. Here are some of our All-American, favorite recipes for breakfast, lunch, and dinner, as well as some of our favorite food products to get you started.

Join the Breakfast Club

It's true: breakfast is the most important meal of the day. So friends, let's make it count and start the day off right. From savory to sweet, here's a selection of our breakfast favorites.

All-American Tofu Scramble

Who said we had to give up our breakfast staples? We can make them more nutritious instead. This breakfast scramble will have you jumping out of bed. Who needs coffee?

Ingredients:

 1 block firm or extra-firm, organic, non-GMO tofu (our favorite brands are Westwood and Nasoya)

 ¼ sweet yellow onion, sliced

5 cloves garlic, crushed

1 tablespoon of soy sauce or tamari sauce

¼ teaspoon turmeric

5 tablespoons nutritional yeast (this gives it that cheesy flavor!)

4 ounces grated, vegan-cheddar cheese (We love the Daiya brand. Pour at your discretion.)

1 carton sliced, button mushrooms

2 cups fresh spinach leaves

⅓ tablespoon of vegan butter (Optional)

Salt and pepper to taste

Fry onion and sliced mushrooms in a little vegan butter (or, for a healthier option, in a little water) until soft and mushrooms are cooked through. Lightly press tofu as you want to retain moisture. In a large bowl, crumble tofu and then add garlic, vegan cheese, nutritional yeast, soy or tamari sauce, turmeric, salt, and pepper. Mix well using a spoon or your hands. Don't be afraid to get down and dirty! Add to onion and mushroom mixture. Cook, stirring occasionally, until cheese has melted and mixture is cooked through. Add spinach and cook until spinach is slightly wilted. Serve immediately.

Make it a meal. Pair this tofu scramble with Lightlife's Smart Bacon, Field Roast Smoked Apple Sage vegan sausages, grilled tomatoes, or whole wheat toast.

Delicious and Nutritious Green Juice

They might be the newest diet trend, but green juices are filled with antioxidants, anti-inflammatory agents, and phytonutrients that will keep you energized and radiating from the inside out. Want to be the cool kid? Get into juicing.

Ingredients:

1 organic kale leaf

Half an organic cucumber

A few pieces of organic pineapple

1 organic apple or pear

A splash of soymilk or water, if you want to make it smoother

Simply blend in a Vitamix or juicer, pour, and top with some ground, organic hemp or flaxseeds for omega-3s.

Perfect Sunday Brunch Blueberry Pancakes

Sunday mornings are made complete with this steaming stack of freshly made pancakes adapted from Isa Chandra Moskowitz's Isa Does It. *While pancakes aren't exactly a health food, blueberries are packed with antioxidants and anti-inflammatories. These are so good you can have them for dinner too. We wouldn't judge you.*

Ingredients:
  1½ cups all-purpose flour
  3½ teaspoons baking powder
  2 tablespoons granulated sugar
  1 cup almond or soy milk (or your favorite nondairy milk)
  2 teaspoons apple cider vinegar
  1 tablespoon ground flaxseed
  ½ cup water
  3 tablespoons canola oil
  ½ teaspoon vanilla extract
  2 teaspoons of vegan butter
  ½ cup of blueberries (Be sure to buy organic berries. Conventional berries are contaminated with pesticides and fertilizers.)

Tricks of the Trade: Use a dinner fork rather than an electric mixer for the batter. Over mixing can result in a dense pancake.

Preheat the pan for a good ten minutes with just a little vegan butter.

In a large bowl, sift together the flour, baking powder, salt, and sugar. Make a well in the center.

Measure the milk into a large measuring cup or small bowl. Add the vinegar and ground flaxseed, and use a fork to vigorously mix the ingredients until foamy. This will take a minute or so.

Pour the milk mixture into the center of the dry ingredients. Add the water, canola oil, and vanilla, and use a fork to mix until a thick, lumpy batter forms for about a minute. It doesn't need to be smooth; just make sure you get all the ingredients incorporated. Pour in the blueberries and mix throughout. Do not overmix.

Use a measuring cup (about ¼ or $^1/_3$ cup) to scoop out the batter for uniformly sized pancakes. Cook for about four minutes until puffy. Flip the pancakes, adding more vegan butter to the pan if needed, and cook for another few minutes.. The pancakes should be a little under an inch thick and golden brown.

Let the pancakes rest on a cooling rack covered with aluminum foil until ready to serve. Top with Earth Balance vegan butter, whipped cashew cream, or organic maple syrup. You can't go wrong. Stack 'em up and enjoy!

Still want that homemade pancake taste without making it from scratch? Cherrybrook Kitchen Original Pancakes™ are our go-to pancake staple. All you need on hand is some soy, almond, or rice milk, and vegetable oil!

Pressed for time? Here are some on-the-go breakfast staples:

1. Engine 2 Diet cereals with blueberries, bananas, and other fruit of your choice and almond, soy, hemp, oat, coconut, or rice milk
2. Fresh fruit. So many options, so little time.
3. Cliff Bars (make sure they are vegan! Some have dairy in them.)
4. Luna Bars
5. Bagels, toast, and muffins

Let's Lunch

Don't skimp on lunch, friends. Our bodies need nourishment throughout the day. What makes the best lunches? Leftovers. See our dinner options. Here are some other, easy lunch options that won't take too much time or energy.

Salads Aren't Boring

Although many people tend to think that vegans live on salads, roasted veggies, and apples, this is not true at all. But we do like our salads. Feel free to put in all of your favorites to make a delicious, healthy salad. Get creative! Here is one of our favorite combinations:

Mixed greens, kale, sliced red cabbage, carrot strips, raw thinly sliced beets, bok choy, cucumber, sliced baby tomatoes, organic cranberries, and toasted walnuts. Other ideas: add avocado, grilled tofu slices, olives, roasted Brussels sprouts, or grilled Beyond Meat Chicken.

Plate your salad, starting with the greens, grouping the colored veggies, and finishing with the red cabbage, cranberries, and walnuts. Add a salad dressing of your choice or top with hummus. Our favorite is SASS Sesame Garlic dressing, found at Whole Foods.

Everything Burritos and Tacos
Mexican food is always a good idea and one of our favorite quick and easy lunches or dinners.

Add any or all of the following to a burrito or a hard-taco shell. Engine 2 or sprouted-grain tortillas are the healthiest.

- Veggie meat sauce with preferred vegan taco seasoning
- Daiya, Follow Your Heart, or Tofutti sour cream
- Refried beans
- Beans and rice
- Chopped tomato and onions
- Guacamole—you can buy vegan guacamole or make your own
- Chopped iceberg lettuce (or spinach as a healthier option)
- Vegan grated cheese

Brown-Bag Sandwich Ideas
Your child's lunch doesn't need to be a tragedy. Here are easy sandwich ideas. There is something for every preference.

The Classic PB&J: Slather peanut butter on whole-wheat bread. Toast it. Want to spice it up? Add sliced bananas.

The Fake Out: From Italian to oven-roasted, Tofurky has enough types to fill your alternative "meat" sandwiches. Add sliced tomato, mustard, Vegenaise spread, hummus, lettuce, or pickles on whole-wheat bread.

The Salad Sandwich: Top any bagel with one of these three salad options: Chick'n, No Tuna, and No Egg.

Old Fashioned Grilled Cheese: Spread vegan butter and Vegenaise on both sides of whole wheat bread. Add Daiya Mozzarella and Cheddar slices or shreds. Sprinkle with Oregano. Grill on both sides. Serve warm!

Plant-Powered Food: It's What's for Dinner

These tried-and-true, healthy and hearty meals are a wonderful start to your plant-powered journey. From Thai stew to mushroom burgers, we have every cuisine to satisfy your palate. Don't take our word for it. Try them for dinner tonight!

Finger-lickin' "Chick'n" Pot Pie

A classic that is perfect for cold, winter nights. This "chick'n" pot pie is sure to impress family and friends. This is made to share, so bring it to your next family weekend or host a dinner party.

Ingredients:

> 2 tablespoons olive oil (sauté in water for a healthier option)
> 1 medium yellow onion, diced
> 1 teaspoon salt (optional)
> ¾ cup peeled carrots, diced into ½-inch pieces
> 2 ribs celery diced into ½-inch pieces
> 4 cloves garlic
> 2 tablespoons fresh thyme
> 2 teaspoons dried, rubbed sage
> 3 tablespoons sherry or white wine
> Several pinches of freshly ground black pepper
> 2 medium russet potatoes, peeled and diced into ½-inch pieces
> 3 cups vegetable broth
> ¼ cup all-purpose flour
> 1 cup water
> ¼–½ packet Beyond Meat chicken strips (or soy vegan nuggets from Delight), diced into ½-inch pieces
> ½ cup frozen peas
> Pepperidge Farm puff pastry

Preheat the oven to 400 degrees Fahrenheit.

For the filling:

Heat a large, cast-iron or oven-safe pan over medium-high heat and add the oil or water. Sauté the onions in the oil or water with a pinch of salt (optional) until softened, about three minutes.

Add the carrots and celery, and sauté for about five more minutes until the onions are lightly browned. Add the garlic, thyme, and sage (crushed in your fingers). Sauté for a minute or so, then add the sherry to deglaze the pan, along with the remaining one teaspoon of salt and the pepper. Let the sherry reduce for a few minutes.

Now add the potatoes and vegetable broth. Cover the pan and bring to a boil. Once boiling, lower the heat and let simmer until the potatoes are tender, about five minutes. Be careful not to overcook them; no one wants mushy potatoes.

In a measuring cup, mix the flour into the water with a fork until no lumps are left. Slowly add the water-flour mixture to the pot, mixing well. Let thicken for five minutes or so. Add the Beyond Meat chicken (or soy nuggets) and peas, and continue to cook. After about five more minutes, it should be perfectly thick but still smooth. Taste for seasoning.

To make the crust:

While the oven is preheating and the stew is thickening, prepare the dough as per the instructions on the box. Gently roll out one of the dough sheets onto a lightly floured surface.

Place a large coffee mug into the center of a casserole dish to keep the dough from collapsing. When the stew is ready, pour into the casserole dish, and smooth with a spatula. Gently place the pastry over the stew. Using a sharp knife, make five, three-inch slits from the center of the casserole to allow the air to escape. Brush top of pastry with water. Place in the oven, and bake for about twenty-five minutes until lightly browned. Remove from oven.

Make it a meal. Serve with a nice green salad and mashed potatoes.

Mamma Goodman's Cottage Pie

Hearty, healthy, and homemade, this secret family recipe comes to you all the way from South Africa. It's a tried-and-true favorite and one of the best comfort foods. We promise you will be coming back for seconds.

Ingredients:

- 1 packet veggie-meat crumbles (Lightlife, Tofurky, or Gardein brands)
- 6 garlic cloves
- 1 yellow onion
- 1 teaspoon mustard powder
- 1 carton sliced, button mushrooms
- 1 can peeled tomatoes
- 1 tin tomato puree
- 2 teaspoons mixed herbs
- 2 teaspoons oregano
- 2 tablespoons vegan Worcestershire sauce
- 1 bay leaf
- About six large potatoes (one bag of small potatoes)
- Vegan butter
- ¼ cup plain almond (or soy, rice, or any other plain-plant) milk
- 2 tablespoons vegan butter
- 1 tablespoon Vegenaise
- Garlic salt, salt, and pepper to taste

Preheat oven to 350 degrees Fahrenheit.

For the filling:

Brown chopped onions in a little olive oil or water. Add garlic and stir for thirty seconds. Add the veggie meat crumbles and brown. Add canned tomatoes, tomato puree, herbs, oregano, mustard, Worcestershire sauce, bay leaf, and freshly sliced, button mushrooms. Simmer for about an hour.

For the mashed potatoes:

Peel and quarter potatoes, and boil until tender. Mash with the soy milk, vegan butter, vegan sour cream, and Vegenaise until creamy. Don't be shy. Add heaping spoonfuls of vegan butter, sour cream, and Vegenaise, and taste test to find what works for you. Spice with garlic powder and pepper.

Putting it all together:

Remove the bay leaf from the sauce. Place the "meat" sauce in a casserole dish and the mashed potatoes on top. Lightly spread some vegan butter on top. Sprinkle paprika, and bake at 350 degrees for thirty minutes or until the potato is slightly crisp on top.

Thai Curry Stew

We win over hearts and minds in favor of plant-powered diets with this simple Thai curry stew, adapted from Skinny Bitch Ultimate Everyday Cookbook *by Kim Barnouin. We promise guests will be begging for more. If there are leftovers, it tastes even better the next day for lunch!*

Ingredients:

2 tablespoons organic canola oil
1 teaspoon ginger
4 garlic cloves, chopped
2 cans organic-coconut milk (14-ounce cans)
1½ cups of water
4+ teaspoons red curry paste
3 tablespoons white-miso paste
3 teaspoons curry powder
1 packet Delight Soy Patties
1 packet organic mushrooms, sliced (we usually use Bella)
1–2 organic carrots, diced
2–3 potatoes, cut into pieces
1–1¼ cup organic frozen broccoli florets
1–2 cups fresh spinach leaves.
Sriracha sauce (to taste)

Heat one tablespoon of oil in a medium frying pan over medium-high heat, and fry soy patties until nicely browned on each side. Remove from pan, and slice into bite-sized pieces. Fry mushrooms until cooked through. Remove from pan.

Heat remaining tablespoon of oil in a large saucepan over medium heat. Add the ginger and garlic, and sauté for fifteen seconds. Add the coconut milk, water, red curry paste, miso paste, and curry powder, and stir until well combined. Reduce the heat to low, and simmer for twenty minutes.

Fill a saucepan halfway with water, and boil quartered potatoes until soft, but don't overcook. Drain.

Add the soy nuggets, mushrooms, and carrots, and simmer for about twenty minutes. Squeeze in four to six drops of Sriracha sauce, or more if you like your curry very strong. Add potatoes and broccoli. Adjust seasonings. Before serving, add one to two cups of spinach leaves, and mix well.

Make it a meal, and serve over Thai jasmine rice.

Mushroom Pecan Burgers (Mmmm-Mmm Good!)
Even those who don't fancy mushrooms will fall in LOVE with these burgers!

Ingredients:
  1½ pounds cremini mushrooms
  1 cup fresh parsley or cilantro
  1 cup cannellini beans
  2 tablespoons olive oil
  2 large-size yellow onions, finely chopped
  4 garlic cloves, minced
  1½–2 cups bread crumbs or cracker meal
  3½ tablepoons plant-based barbecue sauce
  1 cup toasted pecans or walnuts, well chopped
  3 tablespoons tamari soy sauce
  2 teaspoons dried oregano
  ½ teaspoon dried sage
  1 teaspoon thyme
  Salt and ground pepper

In a sauté pan over medium heat, cook onions and garlic for five to six minutes. Place the mixture in a large bowl. Add the minced mushrooms, cilantro or parsley, bread crumbs, barbecue sauce, tahini, chopped nuts, tamari, tyme, oregano, sage, salt, and pepper.

Place the mixture in the refrigerator for about an hour. Form the patties with your hands. The texture will be soft, so add bread crumbs if needed.

In a sauté pan, warm the olive oil, and fry these awesome patties over medium heat for about three or four minutes on each side, until slightly browned and crispy.

Yields ten to twelve servings. You can also put the mixture into a 5" x 9" x 2" loaf pan and bake at 350 degrees Fahrenheit for twenty to twenty-five minutes.

Pâté: Walnut and Mushrooms

We have made this over twenty times and like to play with it, adding and subtracting the personal favorite flavors of the evening's guests. It is adapted from one of our favorite cookbooks, Veganomican. *Whether you want to increase the thyme and tarragon or add sage or black olives, this pate recipe is the best . . . ever. And no rotting, infected liver goes into it!*

Ingredients:
- 4 tablespoons olive oil
- 1 cup diced, yellow onion
- 3 cloves garlic
- 3 teaspoons dried thyme or 9 teaspoons fresh
- 2 teaspoons dried tarragon or 6 teaspoons fresh
- 2 teaspoons dried sage or 6 teaspoons fresh
- 1 teaspoon salt
- Freshly ground black pepper
- 1 pound of your favorite mushrooms, chopped
- 1 cup toasted walnuts
- 1 cup cooked cannellini beans
- ½ cup hummus
- 3 teaspoons balsamic vinegar
- ⅛ cup vegetable broth

Cook onions in a sauté skillet for about four minutes until translucent. Add garlic, thyme, tarragon, sage, salt, and pepper, and cook for another minute. Then add the mushrooms, and cook for another four minutes at medium temperature. Place the walnuts in a food processor or blender and process until very fine.

Add the cooked-mushroom mixture to the walnuts in the food processor. Add the balsamic vinegar, beans, and olive oil. Process until smooth, adding the vegetable broth a little at a time, as needed. Puree the ingredients until the pâté is a thick spread. Scrape mixture into a container, and chill for at least one hour. Bon Appetit!

Yields about 2½ cups.

Delicious White Sauce

This white sauce is quick, easy, and absolutely our favorite sauce to eat with everything. It can be served over roasted vegetables or tofu with rice, or even used as a fettuccine alfredo sauce.

Ingredients:

¼ cup almond oil

1¼ cup water

One package firm, organic tofu (rinsed)

¼ cup Bragg Liquid Aminos

¼ cup Nutritional Yeast Flakes (available at Whole Foods and most health-food stores)

¼ teaspoon kelp powder

¼ teaspoon Spike seasoning (optional)

½ teaspoon organic basil

¼ teaspoon organic, granulated garlic flakes or one or two cloves fresh garlic, depending on your taste

2 tablespoon fresh lemon juice (can use organic bottled)

1 tablespoon Tamari sauce

Blend above ingredients until smooth and creamy. Gently heat in a saucepan on low heat before putting on vegetables or pasta. Store any leftover sauce in the refrigerator.

Let's Celebrate with Dessert!

There are plenty of amazing, melt-in-your-mouth vegan desserts. No, you don't need milk and dairy products to achieve that delicious, sweet satisfaction.

We are the first to admit dessert is not healthy, but fine on occasion. Here are two recipes to enjoy and celebrate your new, compassionate lifestyle!

Vegan Coconut Macaroons
Bet you can't eat just one of these bite-sized delicacies...

Ingredients:
- ⅞ cup sugar, preferably coconut sugar
- ½ cup non-dairy milk
- 5 teaspoons vanilla extract
- ¾ teaspoon salt
- ¾ cup all-purpose flour
- 3 cups unsweetened, shredded coconut

Preheat oven to 350 degrees Fahrenheit.

Mix the sugar, non-dairy milk, vanilla extract, and salt. Blend. Add the coconut and blend well. Then add the flour and mix well. With your hands, form the dough into balls, and place on a lightly oiled cookie tray. These will not change size when heated, so make them to your preference. We prefer about one-inch-all-round balls.

Bake for about twelve to thirteen minutes. Store macaroons in a covered container or freeze in freezer bag or container. Enjoy!

Vegan Chocolate Brandy Cake
Get ready for this cake to rock your world. Adapted from a homemade South African recipe, this cake really does melt in your mouth. It is the perfect cake for birthdays, family gatherings, and gaining popularity among friends.

Chocolate Cake Ingredients:
- 1 cup organic all-purpose flour
- 1 cup organic sugar
- 2 teaspoon baking powder
- ¼ cup cocoa powder
- ½ cup hot water
- ½ cup sunflower (or canola) oil

Ener-G Egg Replacer: Mix 6 teaspoons Ener-G replacer with eight tablespoons water

Non-dairy butter (for cake pan)

Heat oven to 350 degrees Fahrenheit.

Prepare a bundt cake pan using non-dairy butter and flour. We like to use a springform pan.

In a large bowl, sieve together the flour, sugar, and baking powder. Form a hole in the middle of the mixture, and mix in the cocoa powder, hot water, and sunflower (or canola) oil. Mix together until sugar is dissolved.

Beat egg-replacer mixture. Fold the egg replacer into batter.

Bake for about 25 mins. This cake is moist, so be careful not to overbake.

For the Brandy glaze:

½ cup of sugar

½ carton of soy creamer

2 tablespoons of brandy

In a saucepan add the sugar, brandy, and soy creamer, and bring to a boil. Be sure to poke some small holes in the top of the cake so the brandy seeps through. Pour mixture directly over warm cake when removed from oven and still in the pan. Leave to cool.

For the Chocolate Glaze Frosting:

½ bag of non-dairy chocolate chips.

¼ cup of almond (soy, or other plant milk of your choice—although rice milk is far thinner than other plant milks)

Melt the chocolate with the soymilk in a saucepan, stirring frequently. Place the cake onto a plate. Pour the chocolate glaze over the cake, and allow it to set. Serve and enjoy!

Be sure to check out our list of cookbooks and resources to keep your palate sizzling!

Recommended Resources for a Healthy, Happy Life

Want to learn more? Need some inspirational recipe ideas to get started? Want to get in shape? Want to know how to disease-proof your life? Don't worry; we've got you covered. These books, movies, and online resources will keep you connected, informed, inspired, and motivated.

A Cookbook for Every Occasion

There is no shortage of delicious recipe books that don't contain all the crap! From meat substitutes to raw desserts, gorgeous salads, hearty stews, and comfort favorites, these cookbooks can teach you how to make it all.

1. *Artisan Vegan Cheese* by Miyoko Schinner
2. *Betty Goes Vegan* by Annie and Dan Shannon
3. *Chloe's Kitchen* and *Chloe's Vegan Desserts* by Chloe Coscarelli
4. *Crazy Sexy Diet* by Kris Carr
5. *Eat Vegan on $4 a Day* by Ellen Jaffe Jones
6. *Skinny Bitch: Ultimate Everyday Cookbook* by Kim Barnouin

7. *The Candle Café Cookbook* by Joy Pierson, Bart Potenza, and Barbara Scott-Goodman
8. *The Cheesy Vegan* by John Schlimm
9. *Isa Does It* by Isa Chandra Moskowitz
10. *Mayim's Vegan Table* by Mayim Bialik with Jay Gordon
11. *Skinny Bitch Bakery* by Kim Barnouin
12. *Skinny Bitch in the Kitch* by Rory Freedman and Kim Barnouin
13. *The Conscious Cook* by Tal Ronnen
14. *The Happy Herbivore Cookbook* by Lindsay S. Nixon
15. *The Joy of Vegan Baking* and *The Vegan Table* by Colleen Patrick-Goudreau
16. *The Kind Diet* by Alicia Silverstone
17. *The Sublime Restaurant Cookbook* by Nanci Alexander
18. *Unprocessed* by Chef AJ and Glen Merzer
19. *Veganomicon* by Isa Chandra Moskowitz and Terry Hope Romero
20. *Vegan A La Mode* by Hannah Kaminsky
21. *Vegan Chocolate* by Fran Costigan
22. *Vegan Cooking for Carnivores* by Roberto Martin
23. *Vegan Cupcakes Take Over the World* and *Vegan Cookies Invade Your Cookie Jar* by Isa Chandra Moskowitz and Terry Hope Romero
24. *Vegan Diner* by Julie Hasson
25. *Vegan for Life* by Jack Norris and Virginia Messina
26. *Vegan Holiday Kitchen* by Nava Atlas and Susan Voisin
27. *Vegan Soul Kitchen* by Bryant Terry

Stay Classy, Stay Informed

1. *Animal Factory* by David Kirby
2. *Comfortably Unaware* and *Food Choice and Sustainability* by Dr. Richard Oppenlander
3. *Diet for a Small Planet* by Francis Moore Lappe
4. *Dominion* by Matthew Scully

5. *Eating Animals* by Jonathon Safran Foer
6. *Farm Sanctuary* by Gene Baur
7. *Fast Food Nation* by Eric Schlosser
8. *Food Politics* by Marion Nestle
9. *Gristle* by Moby with Miyun Park
10. *High Steaks* by Eleanor Boyle
11. *In Defense of Food* and *The Omnivore's Dilemma* by Michael Pollan
12. *Mad Cowboy* and *No More Bull* by Howard F. Lyman, Glen Merzer, and Joanna Samorow-Merzer
13. *Making a Killing* by Bob Torres
14. *Making Kind Choices* by Ingrid Newkirk
15. *Meat Market* by Erik Marcus
16. *Meatonomics* by David Robinson Simon
17. *Milk: The Deadly Poison* by Robert Cohen
18. *On Being Vegan* by Colleen Patrick-Goudreaux
19. *Pandora's Lunchbox* by Melanie Warner
20. *Righteous Porkchop* by Nicolette Hahn Niman
21. *Skinny Bitch* and *Skinny Bastard* by Rory Freedman and Kim Barnouin
22. *Silent Spring* by Rachel Carson
23. *Slaughterhouse* by Gail A. Eisnitz
24. *The CAFO Reader* edited by Daniel Imhoff
25. *The End of Food* by Paul Roberts
26. *The Engine 2 Diet* and *My Beef with Meat* by Rip Esselstyn
27. *The Food Revolution, Diet for a New America,* and *Voices of the Food Revolution* by John Robbins
28. *The Unhealthy Truth* by Robyn O'Brien and Rachel Kranz
29. *The Vegucation of Robin* by Robin Quivers
30. *The Way We Eat* by Peter Singer and Jim Mason
31. *The World Peace Diet* by Will Tuttle
32. *Veganist* by Kathy Freston
33. *Whole* by Dr. T. Colin Campbell and Howard Jacobson
34. *Why We Love Dogs, Eat Pigs, and Wear Cows* by Melanie Joy, PhD

Get Healthy, Get Fit

1. *Rethink Food: 100+ Doctors Can't Be Wrong* by Shushana Castle and Amy-Lee Goodman
2. *Animals and Public Health* by Aysha Akhtar
3. *Eat and Run* by Scott Jurek
4. *Eat to Live* and *Disease-Proof Your Child* by Dr. Joel Fuhrman
5. *Finding Ultra* by Rich Roll
6. *The Food Prescription for Better Health* by Dr. Baxter D. Montgomery
7. *Healthy Eating for Life for Children* by Physicians Committee for Responsible Medicine and Dr. Amy Lanou
8. *Health Power* by Dr. Hans Diehl and Aileen Ludington
9. *The Whole Heart Solution* by Dr. Joel K. Kahn
10. *Just be Well* by Dr. Thomas A. Sult
11. *Pet Goats and Pap Smears* by Dr. Pamela Wible
12. *The Pillars of Health* by John Pierre
13. *Power Foods for the Brain* and *21-Day Weight Loss Kickstart* by Dr. Neal Barnard
14. *Prevent and Reverse Heart Disease* by Dr. Caldwell B. Esselstyn, Jr.
15. *The China Study* by Dr. T. Colin Campbell with Thomas M. Campbell II
16. *The Expert's Guide to Weight-Loss Surgery* by Dr. Garth Davis and Laura Tucker
17. *The No-Dairy Breast Cancer Prevention Program* and *Your Life in Your Hands* by Prof. Jane Plant
18. *The Starch Solution* by John and Mary McDougall
19. *The Thrive Diet* by Brendan Brazier
20. *Vegan for Her* by Virginia Messina and JL Fields
21. *Vegan for Life* by Jack Norris and Virginia Messina
22. *Waist Away* by Drs. Mary Clifton and Chelsea Clinton
23. *Whitewash* by Joseph Keon

Google These Websites:

1. www.rethinkfoodbook.com
2. www.forksoverknives.com
3. www.engine2diet.com
4. www.ewg.org
5. www.foodsafetynews.com
6. www.foodandwaterwatch.org
7. www.humanesociety.org
8. www.nutritionfacts.org
9. www.pcrm.org
10. www.peta.org
11. www.realfoodchallenge.org
12. www.ucsusa.org
13. www.vegnews.com

Make It a Movie Night

1. *An Inconvenient Truth*
2. *Blackfish*
3. *Earthlings*
4. *Eating*
5. *Fat, Sick, & Nearly Dead*
6. *Food, Inc.*
7. *Food Matters*
8. *Forks Over Knives*
9. *King Corn*
10. *Planeat*
11. *Super Size Me*
12. *Tapped*
13. *The Eleventh Hour*
14. *The Cove*
15. *Vegucated*

REFERENCES

Chapter One:

1 Food and Water Watch, *Factory Farm Nation: How America Turned Its Livestock Farms into Factories* (Washington DC: Food and Water Watch, 2010), 1.

2 Daniel Imhoff, *The CAFO Reader: Tragedy of Industrial Animal Production* (California: Foundation for Deep Ecology, 2010).

3 Pew Commission on Industrial Farm Animal Production, *Putting Meat on the Table: Industrial Farm Animal Production in America* (Maryland: John Hopkins Bloomberg School of Public Health: 2009).

4 James Pearce, "Brave New Jungle: Factory Farming and Advocacy in the Twenty-First Century," *Duke Environmental Law & Policy Forum* 21(2011), 434.

5 Barry Shlachter, "Contract growers hoping the chicken industry offers a steady nest egg may instead be trapped by debt," *Rodale Institute,* 6 March 2005, http://www.newfarm.org/news/2005/0405/040505/contracts.shtml.

6 Eric Schlosser, *Fast Food Nation: The Dark Side of the All-American Meal* (New York: First Mariner Books, 2001): 138.

7	Eric Schlosser, *Fast Food Nation: The Dark Side of the All-American Meal:* 138.

8	Eric Schlosser, *Fast Food Nation: The Dark Side of the All-American Meal:* 138.

9	Renee Johnson, *Recent Acquisitions in Livestock Industry* (Congressional Report, 2009).

10	Food and Water Watch, *Economic Cost of Food Monopolies* (Washington DC: Food and Water Watch, November 2012) https://www.foodandwaterwatch.org/reports/the-economic-cost-of-food-monopolies/.

11	Dan Flynn, "Monopoly Practices Divide Rural America," Food Safety News, 30 August 2010, http://www.foodsafetynews.com/2010/08/monopoly-practices-divide-rural-america/#.U2pu-1d1App. USDA, GIPSA, *Enforcement of the Packers and Stockyards Act,* 2010, (Office of Information and Regulatory Affairs) (9 CFR 201).

12	Christopher Leonard, "USDA Proposes Tougher Meat Industry Anti-Trust Rules," *Huffington Post* 18 June 2010. http://www.huffingtonpost.com/2010/06/18/usda-meat-industry-antitrust_n_618084.html.

13	Christopher Leonard, "USDA Proposes Tougher Meat Industry Anti-Trust Rules," *Huffington Post* 18 June 2010. http://www.huffingtonpost.com/2010/06/18/usda-meat-industry-antitrust_n_618084.html.

14	Congressional Research Service, "USDA's 'GIPSA Rule' on Livestock and Poultry Marketing Practices," By Joel Greene, R41673 (Washington DC, 2014) http://nationalaglawcenter.org/wp-content/uploads/assets/crs/R41673.pdf.

15	Nicolette Hahn Niman, *Righteous Porkchop: Finding a Life and Good Food Beyond Factory Farming* (New York: Harper, 2010).

16	Daniel Imhoff, *The CAFO Reader: Tragedy of Industrial Animal Production* (California: Foundation for Deep Ecology, 2010).

17	Pew Commission on Industrial Farm Animal Production, *Putting Meat on the Table: Industrial Farm Animal Production in America* (Maryland: John Hopkins Bloomberg School of Public Health: 2009).

18 Jeffrey Moussaieff Masson, *The Face on Your Plate: The Truth About Food* (New York: W.W. Norton & Company, 2009).

19 Pew Commission on Industrial Farm Animal Production, *Putting Meat on the Table: Industrial Farm Animal Production in America* (Maryland: John Hopkins Bloomberg School of Public Health: 2009).

20 Union of Concerned Scientists, "Prescription for Trouble: Using Antibiotics to Fatten Livestock," Food & Agriculture, <http://www.ucsusa.org/food_and_agriculture/our-failing-food-system/industrial-agriculture/prescription-for-trouble.html.

21 Eric Schlosser, *Fast Food Nation, The Dark Side of the All-American Meal* (New York: First Mariner, 2001), 136.

22 Beth Kowitt, "McDonald's Buying Power," *CNN Money,* published August 23 2011, http://money.cnn.com/galleries/2011/news/companies/1108/gallery.mcdonalds_buying_power.fortune/index.html.

23 *Inside: McDonalds,* directed by Bloomberg (2013; New York, NY, Netflix) DVD.

24 *Inside: McDonalds,* directed by Bloomberg (2013; New York, NY, Netflix) DVD.

25 Paul Solotaroff, "In the Belly of the Beast," *Rolling Stone,* 10 December 2013, http://www.rollingstone.com/feature/belly-beast-meat-factory-farms-animal-activists.

26 Pew Commission on Industrial Farm Animal Production, *Putting Meat on the Table: Industrial Farm Animal Production in America* (Maryland: John Hopkins Bloomberg School of Public Health: 2009).

27 Institute for Agriculture and Trade Policy, "Playing Chicken: Avoiding Arsenic in Your Meat" (Washington DC:IATP, 2006), http://www.iatp.org/files/421_2_80529.pdf.

28 Food and Water Watch, *Factory Farm Nation: How America Turned Its Livestock Farms into Factories* (Washington DC: Food and Water Watch, 2010).

29 Jeffrey Moussaieff Masson, *The Face on Your Plate: The Truth About Food* (New York: W.W. Norton & Company, 2009).

30 "The Welfare of Cows in the Dairy Industry," Humane Society of the United States, accessed January 2014, http://www.humanesociety.org/assets/pdfs/farm/hsus-the-welfare-of-cows-in-the-dairy-industry.pdf.

31 Joseph Keon, *WhiteWash: The Disturbing Truth About Cow's Milk and Your Health* (Canada: New Society Publishers, 2010).

32 Joseph Keon, *WhiteWash: The Disturbing Truth About Cow's Milk and Your Health* (Canada: New Society Publishers, 2010).

33 Food and Water Watch, *Factory Farm Nation: How American Turned Its Livestock Farms into Factories* (Washington DC: Food and Water Watch, 2010).

Chapter Two:

1   "Environment" *Pew Commission on Farm Animal Production,* 2006, http://www.ncifap.org/issues/environment/ (14 January 2014).

2   Paul Solotaroff, "In the Belly of the Beast," *Rolling Stone,* 10 December 2013, http://www.rollingstone.com/feature/belly-beast-meat-factory-farms-animal-activists.

3   Paul Solotaroff, "In the Belly of the Beast," *Rolling Stone,*10 December 2013, http://www.rollingstone.com/feature/belly-beast-meat-factory-farms-animal-activists.

4   Daniel Imhoff, *The CAFO Reader: Tragedy of Industrial Animal Production* (California: Foundation for Deep Ecology, 2010).

5   Food and Water Watch, *Factory Farm Nation: How America Turned Its Livestock Farms into Factories* (Washington DC: Food and Water Watch, 2010), 1.

6   Food and Water Watch, *Factory Farm Nation: How America Turned Its Livestock Farms into Factories* (Washington DC: Food and Water Watch, 2010).

7 Jennifer Sandy, "Factory Farms: A Bad Choice for Rural America," *Forum Journal* 23 (2009), http://www.preservationnation.org/forum/library/public-articles/factory-farms.html.

8 "Facts About Pollution from Livestock Farms," *National Resources Defense Council,* 21 February2013, http://www.nrdc.org/water/pollution/ffarms.asp.

9 Carrie Hribar, *Understanding Concentrated Animal Feeding Operations and Their Impact on Communities* (Bowling Green: Ohio, 2010), 13.

10 Michele Merkel, *Raising a Stink: Air Emissions from Factory Farms* (Environmental Integrity Project, 2002).

11 David Kirby, *Animal Factory: The Looming Threat of Industrial Pig, Dairy, and Poultry Farms to Humans and the Environment* (New York: St. Martin's Press, 2010).

12 Pew Commission on Industrial Farm Animal Production, *Putting Meat on the Table: Industrial Farm Animal Production in America* (Maryland: John Hopkins Bloomberg School of Public Health: 2009).

13 David Kirby, *Animal Factory: The Looming Threat of Industrial Pig, Dairy, and Poultry Farms to Humans and the Environment* (New York: St. Martin's Press, 2010).

14 "Facts About Pollution from Livestock Farms," *National Resources Defense Council,* 21 February2013, http://www.nrdc.org/water/pollution/ffarms.asp.

15 Daniel Imhoff, *The CAFO Reader: Tragedy of Industrial Animal Production* (California: Foundation for Deep Ecology, 2010).

16 Robbin Marks, *Cesspools of Shame: How Factory Farm Lagoons and Sprayfields Threaten Environmental and Public Health* (National Resource Defense Council and Clean Water Network), 3.

17 Robbin Marks, *Cesspools of Shame: How Factory Farm Lagoons and Sprayfields Threaten Environmental and Public Health* (National Resource Defense Council and Clean Water Network), 3.

18 David Kirby, *Animal Factory: The Looming Threat of Industrial Pig, Dairy, and Poultry Farms to Humans and the Environment* (New York: St. Martin's Press, 2010), 55.

19 David Kirby, *Animal Factory: The Looming Threat of Industrial Pig, Dairy, and Poultry Farms to Humans and the Environment* (New York: St. Martin's Press, 2010), 71.

20 Food and Water Watch, *Factory Farm Nation: How America Turned Its Livestock Farms into Factories* (Washington DC: Food and Water Watch, 2010), 11.

21 Food and Water Watch, *Factory Farm Nation: How America Turned Its Livestock Farms into Factories* (Washington DC: Food and Water Watch, 2010), 15.

22 Food and Water Watch, *Factory Farm Nation: How America Turned Its Livestock Farms into Factories* (Washington DC: Food and Water Watch, 2010), 26.

23 Susan Bourrett, *Meat: A Love Story* (New York: Putnam, 2008) 1.

24 Pew Commission on Industrial Farm Animal Production, *Putting Meat on the Table: Industrial Farm Animal Production in America* (Maryland: John Hopkins Bloomberg School of Public Health: 2009).

25 Carrie Hribar, *Understanding Concentrated Animal Feeding Operations and Their Impact on Communities* (Bowling Green: Ohio, 2010) 14.

26 Daniel Imhoff, *The CAFO Reader: Tragedy of Industrial Animal Production* (California: Foundation for Deep Ecology, 2010).

27 *America's Animal Factories: How States Fail to Prevent Pollution from Livestock Waste* (National Resource Defense Council, 1998).

28 Jeff Tietz, "Boss Hog: The Dark Side of America's Top Pork Producer," *Rolling Stone,* December 2006, http://www.rollingstone.com/culture/news/boss-hog-the-dark-side-of-americas-top-pork-producer-20061214.

29 David Kirby, *Animal Factory: The Looming Threat of Industrial Pig, Dairy, and Poultry Farms to Humans and the Environment* (New York: St. Martin's Press, 2010), 84.

30 Carol Hodne, *Concentrating on Clean Water: The Challenge of Concentrated Animal Feeding Operations* (Iowa: Iowa Policy Project, 2005), 15.

31 Pew Commission on Industrial Farm Animal Production, *Putting Meat on the Table: Industrial Farm Animal Production in America* (Maryland: John Hopkins Bloomberg School of Public Health: 2009).

32 Carol Hodne, *Concentrating on Clean Water: The Challenge of Concentrated Animal Feeding Operations* (Iowa: Iowa Policy Project, 2005), 6.

33 "Facts About Pollution from Livestock Farms," *National Resources Defense Council,* 21 February 2013, http://www.nrdc.org/water/pollution/ffarms.asp.

34 Briseis Kilfoy, Yawei Zhang, Yikyung Park, Theodore Holford et al, "Dietary nitrate and nitrite and the risk of thyroid cancer in the NIH-AARP Diet and Health Study," *Int J Cancer* 129(1)(2011), 160–172.

35 Olga V. Naidenko, Craig Cox, and Nils Bruzelius, *Troubled Waters: Farm Pollution Threatens Drinking Water* (Washington DC: Environmental Working Group, 2009), 12.

36 Olga V. Naidenko, Craig Cox, and Nils Bruzelius, *Troubled Waters: Farm Pollution Threatens Drinking Water* (Washington DC: Environmental Working Group, 2009), 22.

37 Travis Madsen and Benjamin Davis(Frontier Group), and Brad Heavner and John Rumpler, Environment America Research & Policy Center, *Growing Influence: The Political Power of Agribusiness and the Fouling of America's Waterways* (Environment America, 2011), 30.

38 David Kirby, *Animal Factory: The Looming Threat of Industrial Pig, Dairy, and Poultry Farms to Humans and the Environment* (New York: St. Martin's Press, 2010), 92.

39 Jeff Tietz, "Boss Hog: The Dark Side of America's Top Pork Producer," *RollingStone,* December 2006, http://www.rollingstone.com/culture/news/boss-hog-the-dark-side-of-americas-top-pork-producer-20061214.

40 David Kirby, *Animal Factory: The Looming Threat of Industrial Pig, Dairy, and Poultry Farms to Humans and the Environment* (New York: St. Martin's Press, 2010), 93.

41   David Kirby, *Animal Factory: The Looming Threat of Industrial Pig, Dairy, and Poultry Farms to Humans and the Environment* (New York: St. Martin's Press, 2010), 95.

42   David Kirby, *Animal Factory: The Looming Threat of Industrial Pig, Dairy, and Poultry Farms to Humans and the Environment* (New York: St. Martin's Press, 2010), 8.

43   Merritt Frey, et al., Spills and Kills: Manure Pollution and America's Livestock Feedlots (Clean Water Network, Izaak Walton League of America and Natural Resources Defense, 2000), 1.

44   Steven Verburg, "Cleanup of Mile Long Manure Spill near Waunakee Expected to be Completed Soon," *Wisconsin State Journal,* 3 December 2013.

45   Lee Bergquist and Kevin Crowe, "Manure Spills in 2013 the Highest in Seven Years Statewide," *Milwaukee Wisconsin Journal Sentinel,* 5 December 2013, http://www.jsonline.com/news/wisconsin/manure-spills-in-2013-the-highest-in-seven-years-statewide-b99157574z1-234701931.html.

46   Lee Bergquist and Kevin Crowe, "Manure Spills in 2013 the Highest in Seven Years Statewide," *Milwaukee Wisconsin Journal Sentinel,* 5 December 2013, http://www.jsonline.com/news/wisconsin/manure-spills-in-2013-the-highest-in-seven-years-statewide-b99157574z1-234701931.html

47   Lee Bergquist and Kevin Crowe, "Manure Spills in 2013 the Highest in Seven Years Statewide," *Milwaukee Wisconsin Journal Sentinel,* 5 December 2013, http://www.jsonline.com/news/wisconsin/manure-spills-in-2013-the-highest-in-seven-years-statewide-b99157574z1-234701931.html.

48   "Chicken Manure Spill Closes Pennsylvania Playground," *USA Today,* 11 September, 2013.

49   "Coalition to Sue Iowa Hog Operation For Multiple Manure Spills," *Public News Service,* 22 November 2013, http://www.publicnewsservice.org/2013-11-22/animal-welfare/coalition-to-sue-iowa-hog-operation-for-multiple-manure-spills/a35833-1.

50 David Sykes, "Re: Notice of Intent to Sue for Violations of the Clean Water Act," 20 November 2013, http://iowacci.org/wp-content/uploads/2013/11/20131120_Maschhoffs-Keosauqua-CWA-NOI_EIP-CCI-HSUS-2.pdf.

51 Matthew Patane, "Iowa Manure Spills Jump 65% in 2013," *The Des Moines Register*, 4 February 2014, http://www.desmoinesregister.com/story/news/2014/02/04/76-manure-spills-documented-in-iowa-in-2013-a-65-jump/5198145/.

52 The Johns Hopkins Center for A Livable Future, *Feed for Food Producing Animals: A Resource on Ingredients, the Industry, and Regulation*, (Baltimore, Maryland: Bloomberg School of Public Health, 2007), 4.

53 U.S. Department of Agriculture Natural Resources Conservation Service and U.S. Environmental Protection Agency, "Unified National Strategy for Animal Feeding Operations," 11 September 1998.

54 Robin Marks, *Cesspools of Shame: How Factory Farm Lagoons and Sprayfields Threaten Environmental and Public Health* (National Resource Defense Council and Clean Water Network).

55 Jeff Tietz, "Boss Hog: The Dark Side of America's Top Pork Producer," *RollingStone*, December 2006, http://www.rollingstone.com/culture/news/boss-hog-the-dark-side-of-americas-top-pork-producer-20061214.

56 Carol Hodne, *Concentrating on Clean Water: The Challenge of Concentrated Animal Feeding Operations* (Iowa: Iowa Policy Project, 2005) 8.

57 Pierre Gerber, Hennin Steinfeld, et al, *Livestock's Long Shadow: Environmental Issues and Options* (Rome: Food and Agricultural Organization of the United Nations, 2007).

58 Jeff Tietz, "Boss Hog: The Dark Side of America's Top Pork Producer," *RollingStone*, December 2006, http://www.rollingstone.com/culture/news/boss-hog-the-dark-side-of-americas-top-pork-producer-20061214.

59 Jeff Tietz, "Boss Hog: The Dark Side of America's Top Pork Producer," *RollingStone,* December 2006, http://www.rollingstone.com/culture/news/boss-hog-the-dark-side-of-americas-top-pork-producer-20061214.

60 Jeff Tietz, "Boss Hog: The Dark Side of America's Top Pork Producer," *RollingStone,* December 2006, http://www.rollingstone.com/culture/news/boss-hog-the-dark-side-of-americas-top-pork-producer-20061214.

61 Burkholder, J. M. and H. B. Glasgow, "Pfiesteria Piscicida and Other Toxic Pfiesteria-like Dinoflagellates: Behavior, Impacts, and Environmental Controls," *Limnology & Oceanography* 42(5)(1997):1052-1075. E. K., Silbergeld, L. Grattan, et al., "Pfiesteria: harmful algal blooms as indicators of human: ecosystem interactions," *Environmental Research* 82(2)(2000), 97–105.

62 *Animal Factories: Pollution and Human Health Threats to Rural Texas* (Consumers Union SWRO, 2000).

63 The Johns Hopkins Center for A Livable Future, *Feed for Food Producing Animals: A Resource on Ingredients, the Industry, and Regulation* (Baltimore, Maryland: Bloomberg School of Public Health, 2007), 4.

64 Travis Madsen and Benjamin Davis(Frontier Group) and Brad Heavner and John Rumpler, Environment America Research & Policy Center, *Growing Influence: The Political Power of Agribusiness and the Fouling of America's Waterways* (Environment America, 2011).

65 Interagency Working Group on Harmful Algae Blooms, Hypoxia, and Human Health, *Scientific Assessment of Hypoxia in US Coastal Waters* (Committee on Environment and Natural Resources: 2010).

66 United States Department of Agriculture, "E.Coli Alive and Well and Probably in a Streambed Near You," *Agricultural Research* (2011).

67 "Clean Water Act," *United States Environmental Protection Agency,* 2 March 2013.

68 "Clean Water Act," *United States Environmental Protection Agency*, 2 March 2013.

69 Anthony Ladd and Bob Edward, "Corporate Swine and Capitalist Pigs: A Decade of Environmental Injustice and Protest in North Carolina," *Social Justice* 29(3) (2002), 26–46.

70 David Farhenthold, "Manure Becomes a Pollutant as Its Volume Grows Unmanageable," *The Washington Post*, 1 March 2010, http://www.washingtonpost.com/wp-dyn/content/article/2010/02/28/AR2010022803978_3.html?sid=ST2010030100323.

71 "Farm Pollution Knocks Chesapeake Bay Out of Balance," *Environmental Working Group*, 7 December 2010, http://www.ewg.org/news/news-releases/2010/12/06/farm-pollution-knocks-chesapeake-bay-out-balance.

72 U.S. Environmental Protection Agency, *FY08 – FY10 Compliance and Enforcement National Priority: Clean Water Act, Wet Weather, Concentrated Animal Feeding Operations (CAFOs)*, (October 2007).

73 Stephanie Page Ogburn, "Milk and Water Don't Mix," *Food and Environment Reporting Network*, 25 November 2011, http://thefern.org/2011/11/milk-and-water-dont-mix/#sthash.tepKGsaZ.dpuf.

74 Shushana Castle and Amy-Lee Goodman, *Rethink Food: 100+ Doctors Can't Be Wrong* (Houston, TX: Two Skirts Productions), 385.

Chapter Three:

1 G Danaei et al., "The Preventable Causes of Death in the US: Comparative Risk Assessment of Dietary, Lifestyle, and Metabolic Risk Factors," *PLOS Med* 6(4)(2009):e1000058.

2 Centers for Disease Control and Prevention, *National diabetes fact sheet 2011* (Atlanta, GA:CDCP, USDHHS, 2012).

3 Gordon Wardlaw and Anne Smith, *Contemporary Nutrition* (McGraw-Hill, 2010),192.

4   David Robinson Simon, *Meatonomics: How the Rigged Economics of Meat and Dairy Make You Consume Too Much and How to Eat Better, Live Longer, and Spend Smarter* (San Francisco: Conari Press, 2013).

5   Shushana Castle and Amy-Lee Goodman, *Rethink Food: 100+ Doctors Can't Be Wrong* (Houston, TX: Two Skirts Productions, 2014), 8.

6   C Erridge, T Attina, CM Spickett, and DJ Webb, "A High Fat Meal Induces Low-grade Endotoxemia: Evidence of a Novel Mechanism of Postprandial Inflammation," *Am J Clin Nutr* 86(5)(2007): 1286-92. RA Vogel, MC Corretti, GD Plotnick, "Effect of a Single High-fat Meal on Endothelial Function in Healthy Subjects," *Am J Cardiol* 79(3) (1997):350-4. SK Rosenkranz, DK Townsend, SE Steffens, CA Harms, "Effects of a High Fat Meal on Pulmonary Function in Healthy Subjects," *Eur J Appl Physiol* 109(3)(2010), 499–506.

7   Nickolas Bakalar, "Risks: More Red Meat, More Mortality," *The New York Times*, 12 March 2012, http://www.nytimes.com/2012/03/13/health/research/red-meat-linked-to-cancer-and-heart-disease.html?_r=0.

8   Baxter Montgomery, *The Food Prescription for Better Health: A Cardiologists Proven Method to Reverse Heart Disease, Diabetes, Obesity, and Other Chronic Illnesses Naturally* (Houston, TX: Delworth Publishing, 2011), 15.

9   Paul Heindrich et al, "Forecasting the Future of Cardiovascular Disease in the United States: A Policy Statement from the American Heart Association," *Circulation* 123(2011), 933–944.

10 R McClelland, K Nasir, M Budoff, R Blumenthal et al., "Arterial Age as a Function of Coronary Artery Calcium (From the Multi-Ethnic Study of Atherosclerosis [MESA])", *Am J Cardiol* 103, (1)(2009), 59–63. doi:10.1016/j.amjcard.2008.08.031. The Multi-Ethnic Study of Atherosclerosis (MESA) is a medical research study involving more than 6,000 men and women from six communities in the United States. MESA is sponsored by the National Heart Lung and Blood Institute of the National Institutes of Health.

11 F Lowry. "Coronary Atherosclerosis Begins at a Young Age," *Medscape*, 5 Jun 2001, http://www.medscape.com/viewarticle/783668.

12   CJ O'Donnell, R Elosua, "Cardiovascular risk factors: Insights from the Framingham Heart Study," *Rev Esp Cardiol* 61(3)(2008), 299–310.

13   Caldwell B. Esselstyn, *Prevent and Reverse Heart Disease: The Revolutionary, Scientifically Proven, Nutrition Based Cure* (New York: Penguin, 2007).

14   P Pekka, P Pirjo, U Ulla, "Influencing Public Nutrition for Non-communicable Disease Prevention: from Community Intervention to National Programme-Experiences from Finland," *Public Health Nutr* (1A)(2002), 245–51.

15   Joseph Keon, *Whitewash: The Disturbing Truth About Cow's Milk and Your Health* (Canada: New Society Publishers, 2010), 57.

16   Kathy Freston, "Can a Plant-Based Diet Cure Cancer? *Oprah Health and Wellness,* 23 October 2009, http://www.oprah.com/health/Can-a-Plant-Based-Diet-Cure-Cancer#ixzz2U7uSKw89. Shushana Castle and Amy-Lee Goodman, "Chapter Nine: Dear Cancer," *Rethink Food: 100+ Doctors Can't Be Wrong,* (Houston, TX: Two Skirts Productions, 2014), 177–202.

17   "Colorectal Cancer: Latest Evidence," *World Cancer Research Fund,* 4 February 2014, http://www.dietandcancerreport.org/cup/current_progress/colorectal_cancer.php.

18   "AICR Statement: Hot Dogs and Cancer Risk," *American Institute for Cancer Research,* 22 July 2009, http://preventcancer.aicr.org/site/News2?page=NewsArticle&id=15642&news_iv_ctrl=0&abbr=pr_.

19   Shushana Castle and Amy-Lee Goodman, *Rethink Food: 100+ Doctors Can't Be Wrong* (Houston, TX: Two Skirts Productions, 2014), 15.

20   Shushana Castle and Amy-Lee Goodman, *Rethink Food: 100+ Doctors Can't Be Wrong* (Houston, TX: Two Skirts Productions, 2014), 15.

21   Shushana Castle and Amy-Lee Goodman, *Rethink Food: 100+ Doctors Can't Be Wrong* (Houston, TX: Two Skirts Productions, 2014), 288.

22   Shushana Castle and Amy-Lee Goodman, *Rethink Food: 100+ Doctors Can't Be Wrong* (Houston, TX: Two Skirts Productions, 2014), 205–210.

23 RJ Barnard, JH Gonzalez, ME Liva, TH Ngo, "Effects of a Low Fat, High Fiber Diet and Exercise Program on Breast Cancer Risk Factors In Vivo and Tumor Cell Growth and Apotosis In Vitro," *Nutr Cancer* 55(1) (2006):28-34. D Ornish, G Weidner, WR Fair, R Marlin, EB Pettengill et al, *"Intensive Lifestyle Changes May Affect the Progression of Prostate Cancer" J Urol* 174(3)(2005), 1065–9.

24 D. Ornish, MJ Magbanua, V Weinberg, C Kemp et al., "Change in Prostate Gene Expression in Men Undergoing an Intensive Nutrition and Lifestyle Intervention," *Proc Natl Acad Sci USA* 105(24)(2008):8369-74. doi:10.1073/pnas.0803080105.

25 Alexandra Sifferlin, "WHO: Annual Cancer Cases To Hit 22 Million," *TIME*, 3 February 2014, http://healthland.time.com/2014/02/03/cancer-cases-to-hit-22-million/?utm_source=Daily+Skimm&utm_campaign=4c85558b08-daily_skimm&utm_medium=email&utm_term=0_74efee6205-4c85558b08-23329457.

26 CC Cowie et al, "Full Accounting of Diabetes and Pre-diabetes in the US Populations from 1988 to 2006," *Diabetes Care* 32(3)(2011), 287–94.

27 William Herman, "The Economic Costs of Diabetes: Is it Time for a New Treatment Paradigm?," *Diabetes Care* 36(2013), 775–776.

28 Steven Reinberg, "US Diabetes Rates Soaring: CDC," *US News Health*, 5 November 2012, http://health.usnews.com/health-news/news/articles/2012/11/15/us-diabetes-rates-soaring-cdc.

29 Shushana Castle and Amy-Lee Goodman, *Rethink Food: 100+ Doctors Can't Be Wrong* (Houston, TX: Two Skirts Productions, 2014), 154–174.

30 Neal Barnard, Joshua Cohen, David Jenkins, Gabrielle Turner-McGrievy et al., "A Low-Fat Vegan Diet Improves Glycemic Control and Cardio-vascular Risk Factors in a Randomized Clinical Trial in Individuals with Type 2 Diabetes," *Diabetes Care* 29(8)(2006), 1777–1783.

31 Sharon Kirkey, "Drinking Milk Not Essential for Humans Despite Belief it Prevents Osteoporosis, Nutritionist says," *National Post,* 23 January 2014, http://life.nationalpost.com/2014/01/23/drinking-milk-not-essential-for-humans-despite-belief-it-prevents-osteoporosis-nutritionist-says/.

32 Justine Butler, *White Lies* (Bristol: Viva! Health, 2006).

33 Dan Buettner, *The Blue Zones: Lessons for Living Longer From the People Who've Lived the Longest* (Washington DC: National Geographic, 2009).

34 MJ Orlich, PN Singh, J Sabati et al, "Vegetarian Dietary Patterns and Mortality in Adventist Health Study 2," *JAMA Intern Med* 173(13) (2013), 1230–8.

35 Congress Senate Selection Committee, "Nutrition and Human Needs: Dietary Goals for the United States, (US Government Print Office, 1977).

36 Rita Cain, "Food, Inglorious Food: Food Safety, Food Libel and Free Speech," *American Business Law Journal* 49(2012).

37 "Meat MythCrushers," February 2014, http://www.meatmythcrushers. com/.

38 "USDA Sued Over Deceptive Language in New Dietary Guidelines," *Alliance for Natural Health,* 22 March 2011, http://www.anh-usa.org/ usda-sued-over-deceptive-language-in-new-dietary-guidelines/.

39 David Robinson Simon, *Meatonomics: How the Rigged Economics of Meat and Dairy Make You Consume Too Much and How to Eat Better, Live Longer, and Spend Smarter* (San Francisco: Conari Press, 2013).

40 "Highlights from the Dairy Checkoff's Annual Meeting," *DairyBusiness,* 16 January 2014, http://dairybusiness.com/dairyline_headline.php? item=Highlights+from+the+Dairy+Checkoff%E2%80%99s+Annual+ Meeting.

41 David Robinson Simon, *Meatonomics: How the Rigged Economics of Meat and Dairy Make You Consume Too Much and How to Eat Better, Live Longer, and Spend Smarter* (San Francisco: Conari Press, 2013), 63.

42 Michele Simon, *And Now a Word From Our Sponsors: Are America's Nutrition Professional in the Pocket of Big Food* (EatDrinkPolitics: 2013). http://www.eatdrinkpolitics.com/wp-content/uploads/AND_Corpo- rate_Sponsorship_Report.pdf.

43   Michele Simon, *And Now a Word From Our Sponsors: Are America's Nutrition Professional in the Pocket of Big Food* (EatDrinkPolitics: 2013). http://www.eatdrinkpolitics.com/wp-content/uploads/AND_Corporate_Sponsorship_Report.pdf.

44   "Health Benefits and Nutrients: Dairy," *USDA,* 16 January 2014, http://www.choosemyplate.gov/food-groups/dairy-why.html.

45   "Health Benefits and Nutrients: Dairy," *USDA,* 16 January 2014, http://www.choosemyplate.gov/food-groups/dairy-why.html.

46   CDC, *The Power of Prevention: Chronic Disease…The Public Health Challenge of the 21st Century* (National Center for Chronic Disease Prevention and Health Promotion, 2009).

47   CDC, *The Power of Prevention: Chronic Disease…The Public Health Challenge of the 21st Century* (National Center for Chronic Disease Prevention and Health Promotion, 2009), 1.

48   David Robinson Simon, *Meatonomics: How the Rigged Economics of Meat and Dairy Make You Consume Too Much and How to Eat Better, Live Longer, and Spend Smarter* (San Francisco: Conari Press, 2013).

Chapter Four:

1   Pink slime for School Lunch: Government Buying 7 Million Pounds of Ammonia Treated Meat for Meals," *Huffington Post,* 5 March 2012, http://www.huffingtonpost.com/2012/03/05/pink-slime-for-school-lun_n_1322325.html.

2   "Pink slime for School Lunch: Government Buying 7 Million Pounds of Ammonia Treated Meat for Meals," *Huffington Post,* 5 March 2012, http://www.huffingtonpost.com/2012/03/05/pink-slime-for-school-lun_n_1322325.html.

3   Rory Freedman and Kim Barnouin, *Skinny Bitch* (Pennsylvania: Running Press, 2005), 108.

4   Neal Barnard, *Power Foods for the Brain: An Effective 3-Step Plan to Protect Your Mind and Strengthen Your Memory* (New York: Grand Central Life and Style, 2009).

5   VJ Koller, M Furhacker, A Nersesyan, M. Misik, et al, "Cytotoxic and
     DNA-Damaging Properties of Glyphosate and Roundup in Human-
     Derived Buccal Epithelial Cells," *Arch Toxicol* 86 (5)(2012):805-13. doi:
     10.1007/s00204-012-0804-8.

6   Brett Blumenthal, "10 Worst Food Additives and Where They Lurk,"
     GAIAM Life, accessed January 2014, http://life.gaiam.com/article/10-
     worst-food-additives-where-they-lurk.

7   Neal Barnard, *Power Foods for the Brain: An Effective 3-Step Plan to
     Protect Your Mind and Strengthen Your Memory* (New York: Grand
     Central Publishing, 2013).

8   David Kirby, "Drugs, Poisons, and Metals in Our Meat—USDA Needs a
     Major Overhaul, *Huffington Post Healthy Living,* 14 April 2010, http://
     www.huffingtonpost.com/david-kirby/
     food-safety----drugs-pois_b_537686.html.

9   America Farm Bureau Federation, "Fast Facts About Agriculture," *The
     Voice of Agriculture,* last modified 2013, http://www.fb.org/index.php/
     index.php?action=newsroom.fastfacts.

10   The Johns Hopkins Center for A Livable Future, *Feed for Food Producing
     Animals: A Resource on Ingredients, the Industry, and Regulation,*
     (Baltimore, Maryland: Bloomberg School of Public Health, 2007).

11   David Robinson Simon, *Meatonomics: How the Rigged Economics of
     Meat and Dairy Make You Consume Too Much and How to Eat Better,
     Live Longer, and Spend Smarter* (San Francisco: Conari Press, 2013).

12   Tom Philpott, "The Meat Industry Now Consumes Four-Fifths of All
     Antibiotics," *MotherJones,* 8 February 2013, http://www.motherjones.com/
     tom-philpott/2013/02/meat-industry-still-gorging-antibiotics.

13   "Saving Antibiotics", *Natural Resources Defense Council,* 7 February
     2014, http://www.nrdc.org/food/saving-antibiotics.asp.

14   Consumer Reports, "What's in that Pork: We Found Antibiotic-
     Resistant Bacteria and Traces of a Veterinary Drug" *Consumer Reports
     Magazine* (January 2013).

15 Helena Bottemiller, "Science on Antibiotic Resistance is Clear," *Food Safety News,* 13 March 2012, http://www.foodsafetynews.com/2012/03/health-advocates-science-on-antibiotic-resistance-is-clear/#.UvaeN-PldWSo.

16 CDC, *Antibiotic Resistance Threats in the United States, 2013,* (United States Department of Health and Human Resources, 2013).

17 Tom Philpott, "The Meat Industry Now Consumes Four-Fifths of All Antibiotics," *MotherJones,*8 February 2013, http://www.motherjones.com/tom-philpott/2013/02/meat-industry-still-gorging-antibiotics.

18 David Pierson, "Poultry Plants Linked to Outbreaks Won't Be Closed, *Los Angeles Times,* 10 October 2013, http://articles.latimes.com/2013/oct/10/news/chi-no-closing-poultry-plants-linked-to-outbreak-20131010/2.

19 David Pierson, "Washing Chicken Can Spread Salmonella," *Los Angeles Times,* 9 October 2013, http://articles.latimes.com/2013/oct/09/business/la-fi-mo-cleaning-chicken-20131009.

20 Consumer Reports, "What's in that Pork: We Found Antibiotic-Resistant Bacteria and Traces of a Veterinary Drug" *Consumer Reports Magazine* (January 2013).

21 Robin Marks, *Cesspools of Shame: How Factory Farm Lagoons and Sprayfields Threaten Environmental and Public Health* (National Resource Defense Council and Clean Water Network).

22 Pew Commission on Industrial Farm Animal Production, *Putting Meat on the Table: Industrial Farm Animal Production in America,* (Maryland: Johns Hopkins Bloomberg School of Public Health: 2009).

23 David Robinson Simon, *Meatonomics: How the Rigged Economics of Meat and Dairy Make You Consume Too Much and How to Eat Better, Live Longer, and Spend Smarter* (San Francisco: Conari Press, 2013), 61.

24 "Rep. Slaughter: Voluntary Regulation on Antibiotics Inadequate To Protect Public Health; No Enforcement Mechanism or Criteria for Success," *Congresswoman Louise Slaughter,* 11 December 2013, http://www.louise.house.gov/press-releases/rep-slaughter-voluntary-

regulation-on-antibiotics-inadequate-to-protect-public-health-no-enforcement-mechanism-or-criteria-for-success/.

25 "Reps. Waxman and Slaughter Introduce Legislation to Better Monitor Antibiotic Use in Animals," *Rep. Henry A Waxman,* 26 February 2013, http://waxman.house.gov/reps-waxman-and-slaughter-introduce-legislation-better-monitor-antibiotic-use-animals.

26 David Pierson, Diana Marcum and Tiffany Hsu, "Poultry Plants Linked to Outbreak Won't be Closed," *Los Angeles Times,* 10 October 2013, http://articles.latimes.com/2013/oct/10/news/chi-no-closing-poultry-plants-linked-to-outbreak-20131010/2.

27 Pew Commission on Industrial Farm Animal Production, *Putting Meat on the Table: Industrial Farm Animal Production in America,* (Maryland: John Hopkins Bloomberg School of Public Health: 2009).

28 Caitlin Taylor, "Obama Administration: Out with the Swine, In with H1N1, *ABC News,* 29 April 2009, http://abcnews.go.com/blogs/politics/2009/04/obama-adminis-5/.

29 David Robinson Simon, *Meatonomics: How the Rigged Economics of Meat and Dairy Make You Consume Too Much and How to Eat Better, Live Longer, and Spend Smarter* (San Francisco: Conari Press, 2013).

30 Andrew Gunther, "Would You Like Extra Ractopamine with Your Pork, Sir?" Huffington Post, 5 December 2012, http://www.huffingtonpost.com/andrew-gunther/would-you-like-extra-ract_b_2206643.html.

31 Food and Water Watch, *Ractopamine: Fact Sheet* (Food and Water Watch, 2013).

32 Ellen Barry, "Russia Announces Barriers on Imports of US Meat," *The New York Times,* 8 December 2012, http://www.nytimes.com/2012/12/09/world/europe/russia-announces-barriers-on-imports-of-us-meat.html.

33 Vladislav Vorotnikov, "Russia Lifts Ban on Imports of Turkey and Beef from USA," *Global Meat News,* 6 November 2013, http://www.globalmeatnews.com/Industry-Markets/Russia-lifts-ban-on-imports-of-turkey-and-beef-from-the-USA.

34 Food and Water Watch, *Ractopamine: Fact Sheet* (Food and Water Watch, 2013).

35 Linda Ly, "FDA Bans Most Arsenic in Chicken Feed-Oh By the Way There's Arsenic in Your Chicken," *KCET,* 9 October 2013, http://www.kcet.org/living/food/the-nosh/commentary-1/fda-finally-bans-most-arsenic-in-chicken-feed-oh-and-by-the-way-theres-arsenic-in-your-chicken.html.

36 Chris Hunt, "The Arsenic in Your Chicken," *Huffington Post Green,* 13 May 2013, http://www.huffingtonpost.com/chris-hunt/arsenic-in-chicken_b_3267334.html.

37 David Kirby, *Animal Factory: The Looming Threat of Industrial Pig, Dairy, and Poultry Farms to Humans and the Environment* (New York: St. Martin's Press, 2010), 381.

38 David Kirby, *Animal Factory: The Looming Threat of Industrial Pig, Dairy, and Poultry Farms to Humans and the Environment* (New York: St. Martin's Press, 2010), 384.

39 David Kirby, *Animal Factory: The Looming Threat of Industrial Pig, Dairy, and Poultry Farms to Humans and the Environment* (New York: St. Martin's Press, 2010), 381.

40 Sabrina Tavernise, "Study Finds an Increase in Arsenic Levels in Chicken, *The New York Times,* 11 May 2013, http://www.nytimes.com/2013/05/11/health/study-finds-an-increase-in-arsenic-levels-in-chicken.html.

41 Chris Hunt, "The Arsenic in Your Chicken," *Huffington Post Green,* 13 May 2013, http://www.huffingtonpost.com/chris-hunt/arsenic-in-chicken_b_3267334.html.

42 David Kirby, *Animal Factory: The Looming Threat of Industrial Pig, Dairy, and Poultry Farms to Humans and the Environment,* (New York: St. Martin's Press, 2010), 381.

43 Chris Hunt, "The Arsenic in Your Chicken," *Huffington Post Green,* 13 May 2013, http://www.huffingtonpost.com/chris-hunt/arsenic-in-chicken_b_3267334.html.

44 James Greiff, "What's Arsenic Doing in Our Chicken, Anyway?,"
    BloombergView, 10 October 2013, http://www.bloomberg.com/
    news/2013-10-10/what-was-arsenic-doing-in-our-chicken-anyway-.
    html.

45 Stephanie Strom, "FDA Bans Three Arsenic Drugs Used in Poultry and
    Pig Feeds," *The New York Times,* 1October 2013, http://www.nytimes.
    com/2013/10/02/business/fda-bans-three-arsenic-drugs-used-in-
    poultry-and-pig-feeds.html?_r=0.

46 Sabrina Tavernise, "Study Finds an Increase in Arsenic Levels in
    Chicken," *The New York Times,*11 May 2013, http://www.nytimes.
    com/2013/05/11/health/study-finds-an-increase-in-arsenic-levels-in-
    chicken.html?_r=0.

47 "Dixons and Furans: The Most Toxic Chemicals Known to Science"
    Energy Justice Network, 1 February 2012, http://www.ejnet.org/dioxin/.

48 United States Department of the Interior, "Environmental Health: Toxic
    Substances," *United States Geologic Survey,* 5 May 2014, http://toxics.
    usgs.gov/definitions/dioxins.html.

49 Sarah Parsons, "Why the US Government Won't Protect Us from Toxic
    Chemicals in Our Food Supply," *GOOD,* 7 February 2012, http://
    magazine.good.is/articles/why-the-u-s-government-won-t-protect-us-
    from-toxic-chemicals-in-our-food-supply.

50 United States Food and Drug Administration, "Questions and Answers
    About Dioxins and Food Safety," *United States Department of Health and
    Human Services,* February 2012, http://www.fda.gov/Food/Foodbor-
    neIllnessContaminants/ChemicalContaminants/ucm077524.htm.

51 "Dixons and Furans: The Most Toxic Chemicals Known to Science"
    Energy Justice Network, 1 February 2012, http://www.ejnet.org/dioxin/.

52 United States Food and Drug Administration, "Questions and Answers
    About Dioxins and Food Safety," *United States Department of Health and
    Human Services,* February 2012, http://www.fda.gov/Food/Foodbor-
    neIllnessContaminants/ChemicalContaminants/ucm077524.htm.

Chapter Five:

1   Susan Bourrett, *Meat: A Love Story* (New York: Putnam, 2008), 26.

2   Nicolette Hahn Niman, *Righteous Porkchop: Finding a Life and Good Food Beyond Factory Farming,* (New York: Harper, 2010), 155.

3   ME. Patrick, BE Mahon, SM Zansky, S Hurd, and E Scallan, "Riding in Shopping Carts and Exposure to Raw Meat and Poultry Products: Prevalence of and Factors Associated with this Risk Factor for Salmonella and Campylobacter Infection in Children Younger than 3 Years," *J Food Prot* 73(6)(2010), 1097–100.

4   Michael Greger MD, "Avoiding Chicken to Avoid Bladder Infections," *NutritionFacts.org,* 10 June 2013, http://nutritionfacts.org/video/avoiding-chicken-to-avoid-bladder-infections/. AR Manges, JR Johnson, "Food-borne Origins of Escherichiacoli Causing Extraintestinal Infections," *Clin Infect Dis* 55(5)(2012), 712–719.

5   "Alex's Story," *STOP Foodborne Illness,* accessed 20 January 2014, http://www.stopfoodborneillness.org/content/alexs-story.

6   Kathy Freston, "E.Coli Salmonella and Other Deadly Bacteria and Pathogens are in Food: Factory Farms Are the Reason," *Huffington Post Books,* 8 January 2010, http://www.huffingtonpost.com/kathy-freston/e-coli-salmonella-and-oth_b_415240.html.

7   "Food Safety Homepage," *Center for Disease Control and Prevention,* http://www.cdc.gov/foodsafety/, 17 April 2014.

8   Andy Frame, "Policy Changes in the Wake of the Jack in the Box E.Coli Outbreak," *Food Safety News,* 1 February 2013, http://www.foodsafetynews.com/2013/02/policy-changes-since-the-jack-in-the-box-e-coli-outbreak/#.UvXmVPldWSp.

9   Andy Frame, "Policy Changes in the Wake of the Jack in the Box E.Coli Outbreak," *Food Safety News,* 1 February 2013, http://www.foodsafetynews.com/2013/02/policy-changes-since-the-jack-in-the-box-e-coli-outbreak/#.UvXmVPldWSp.

10 Mary McKenna, "Big News But: USDA Bans Other E.Coli Strains," *Wired,* 13 September 2011, http://www.wired.com/2011/09/other-e-coli/.

11 Maryn McKenna, "Does Foodborne Illness Trigger Lifelong Health Problems," *Wired,* 30 March 2012, http://www.wired.com/wiredscience/2012/03/foodborne-lifelong-problems/.

12 Eve Conant, "America's Dangerous Food-Safety System," *The Daily Beast,* 11 September 2011, http://www.thedailybeast.com/articles/2011/09/13/food-safety-system-endangers-americans-due-to-lack-of-inspectors-budget-cuts.html.

13 Michael Greger MD, "Chicken Out of UTIs," *NutritionFacts.org,* 14 October 2010, http://nutritionfacts.org/video/chicken-out-of-utis/. X. Xia, J Meng, PF McDermott et al, "Presence and Characterization of Shiga Toxin-Producing Escherichia Coli and Other Potentially Diarrheagenic E.Coli Strains in Retail Meats," *Appl Environ Microbiol* 76(6) (2010), 1709–1717.

14 Michael Greger MD, "Avoiding Chicken to Avoid Bladder Infections," *NutritionFacts.org,* 10 June 2013, http://nutritionfacts.org/video/avoiding-chicken-to-avoid-bladder-infections/. AR Manges, JR Johnson, "Food-Borne Origins of Escherichiacoli Causing Extraintestinal Infections," *Clin Infect Dis* 55(5)(2012), 712–719.

15 "Americans to Consume 1.25 Billion Chicken Wings During SuperBowl, 25 Billion for all of 2012," *Huffington Post Food,* 24 January 2012, http://www.huffingtonpost.com/2012/01/24/americans-chicken-wings_n_1224547.html.

16 Janice Boase, "Notable FoodBorne Illness Outbreaks of 2011," Food Safety News, 30 December 2011, http://www.foodsafetynews.com/2011/12/notable-foodborne-illness-outbreaks-of-2011/#.U2tuOPldWSo.

17 Mary Clare Jalonick, "Egg Recall Expands to More than Half Billion Nationwide," Huffington Post, 20 August 2010, http://www.huffingtonpost.com/2010/08/21/egg-recall-expands-to-mor_n_690019.html.

18 "Multistate Outbreak of Multistate Outbreak of Human *Salmo-nella* Heidelberg Infections Linked to Ground Turkey, *Centers for Disease Control,* 29 September 2011, http://www.cdc.gov/salmonella/heidelberg/092911/.

19 Kathy Freston, "E. Coli, Salmonella and Other Deadly Bacteria and Pathogens in Food: Factory Farms Are the Reason," *Huffington Post,* 8 January 2010, http://www.huffingtonpost.com/kathy-freston/e-coli-salmonella-and-oth_b_415240.html.

20 Kathy Freston, "E. Coli, Salmonella and Other Deadly Bacteria and Pathogens in Food: Factory Farms Are the Reason," *Huffington Post,* 8 January 2010, http://www.huffingtonpost.com/kathy-freston/e-coli-salmonella-and-oth_b_415240.html.

21 Centers for Disease Control and Prevention, *National Antimicrobial Resistance Monitoring System (NARMS): Enteric Bacteria Annual Report* (2009). A. Karapetian, "A Model EU," *Meatingplace* (2010), 91.

22 Michael Greger MD, "Why is Selling Salmonella Tainted Chicken Legal?" *NutritionFacts.org,* 1 October 2013, http://nutritionfacts.org/2013/10/01/why-is-selling-salmonella-tainted-chicken-still-legal/.

23 Michael Greger MD, "Why is Selling Salmonella Tainted Chicken Legal?," *NutritionFacts.org,* 1 October 2013, http://nutritionfacts.org/2013/10/01/why-is-selling-salmonella-tainted-chicken-still-legal/.

24 James Andrews, "Salmonella on Chicken: Is Zero Tolerance Feasible?," *Food Safety News,* 5 February 2014, http://www.foodsafetynews.com/2014/02/is-zero-tolerance-on-salmonella-feasible/#.UvX0dvldWSp.

25 Michael Greger MD, "Why is Selling Salmonella Tainted Chicken Legal?" *NutritionFacts.org,* 1 October 2013, http://nutritionfacts.org/2013/10/01/why-is-selling-salmonella-tainted-chicken-still-legal/.

26 Centers for Disease Control and Prevention, *National Antimicrobial Resistance Monitoring System (NARMS): Enteric Bacteria Annual Report* (2009). A. Karapetian, "A Model EU," *Meatingplace* (2010), 91.

27 "FrontLine Modern Meat: Interview Eric Schlosser," *PBS*, http://www.
    pbs.org/wgbh/pages/frontline/shows/meat/interviews/schlosser.html, 4
    February 2014.

28 Michael Greger MD, "Why is Selling Salmonella Tainted Chicken
    Legal?," *NutritionFacts.org*, 1 October 2013, http://nutritionfacts.
    org/2013/10/01/why-is-selling-salmonella-tainted-chicken-still-legal/.

29 James Andrews, "Salmonella on Chicken: Is Zero Tolerance Feasible?,"
    Food Safety News, 5 February 2014, http://www.foodsafetynews.
    com/2014/02/is-zero-tolerance-on-salmonella-feasible/#.UvX0dvldWSp.

30 CC Tam, LC Rodrigues, I Petersen et al, "Incidence of Guillain-Barre
    Syndrome Among Patients with Campylobacter Infection: A General
    Practice Research Database Study, *Journal Infectious Disease* 194 (2006):
    95-97. TA Hardy, S Blum, PA McCombe, SW Reddel, "Guillian Barre
    Syndrome: Modern Theories of Etiology," *Curr Allergy Asthma Rep*
    11(2011): 197-204. doi: 10.1007/s11882-011-0190-y. N Shahrizalla, N
    Yuki, "The First Proof of Molecular Mimicry in Human Autoimmune
    Disorder" *J Biomed Biotechnol* 2011(2011): 829129. I Nachamkin, BM
    Allos, T Ho, "Campylobacter Species and Guillian- Barre Syndrome,"
    Clin Microbiol Rev 11 (1998), 555–67.

31 The Johns Hopkins Center for A Livable Future, *Feed for Food Producing
    Animals: A Resource on Ingredients, the Industry, and Regulation* (Balti-
    more, Maryland: Bloomberg School of Public Health, 2007).

32 "Mad Cow Disease Fast Facts," *CNN*, 27 September 2013, http://www.
    cnn.com/2013/07/02/health/mad-cow-disease-fast-facts/.

33 Charles Abbott, "Court Bars Meatpacker Tests for Mad Cow," *Reuters*,
    29 August 2008, http://www.reuters.com/article/2008/08/29/us-usa-
    madcow-tests-idUSN2928450820080829.

34 Eric Schlosser, *Fast Food Nation, The Dark Side of the All-American
    Meal* (New York: First Mariner, 2001), 201.

35 Eric Schlosser, *Fast Food Nation, The Dark Side of the All-American
    Meal* (New York: First Mariner, 2001), 202.

36　Eric Schlosser, *Fast Food Nation, The Dark Side of the All-American Meal* (New York: First Mariner, 2001), 201.

37　Jeanine Skowronski, "8 Big Productivity Killers at Work," *Mainstreet*, 24 October 2011, http://www.mainstreet.com/slideshow/career/8-big-productivity-killers-work.

38　James Pearce, "Brave New Jungle: Factory Farming and Advocacy in the Twenty-First Century," *Duke Environmental Law & Policy Forum* 21(2011), 437.

39　Rod Leonard, *Losing Control of Food Safety* (Minneapolis, Minnesota: The Institute for Agriculture and Trade Policy, 2007).

40　GAO, *Meat and Poultry: Better USDA Oversight and Enforcement of Safety Rules Needed to Reduce Risk of Foodborne Illness*, Washington DC: US General Accounting Office, August 2002 (GAO-02-902)(Report to the Committee on Agriculture, Nutrition, Forestry, US Senate) http://www.gao.gov/new.items/d02902.pdf.

41　News Desk, "GAO Report Questions USDA Plans to Change Poultry Inspection Program," *Food Safety News*, 4 September 2013, http://www.foodsafetynews.com/2013/09/gao-report-questions-validity-of-usda-poultry-inspection-plans/#.UvZGIfldWSq.

42　Government Accountability project, "USDA Inspectors: Government 'HIMP' Plan is a Threat to Food Safety," April 2012, http://www.whistle-blower.org/storage/documents/FIC_HIMP_Affidavit_1.pdf.

43　David Dayen, "USDA Seeks to Let Poultry Companies Self-Inspect Their Product," *FDL NewsDesk*, 5 April 2012, http://news.firedoglake.com/2012/04/05/usda-seeks-to-let-poultry-companies-self-inspect-their-product/.

44　United States Government Accountability Office, *Food Safety: More Disclosure and Data Needed to Clarify Impact of Changes to Poultry and Hog Inspections*, Washington DC:US Government Accountability Office, August 2013 (GAO-13-775: USDA Inspection Pilot Programs), (Report to the Chairman, Subcommittee on Livestock, Dairy, Poultry, Marketing and Agriculture Security, Committee on Agriculture, Nutrition and Forestry, US Sentate), http://www.gao.gov/products/GAO-13-775.

45 Eve Conant, "America's Dangerous Food-Safety System," *The Daily Beast*, 11 September 2011, http://www.thedailybeast.com/articles/2011/09/13/food-safety-system-endangers-americans-due-to-lack-of-inspectors-budget-cuts.html.

Chapter Six:

1 Joseph Keon, *Whitewash: The Disturbing Truth About Cow's Milk and Your Health* (Canada: New Society Publishers, 2010) 9.

2 Joseph Keon, *Whitewash: The Disturbing Truth About Cow's Milk and Your Health* (Canada: New Society Publishers, 2010), 5.

3 Joseph Keon, *Whitewash: The Disturbing Truth About Cow's Milk and Your Health* (Canada: New Society Publishers, 2010), 109.

4 John Robbins, No Happy Cow: Dispatches from the Front Lines of the Food Revolution (San Francisco: Conari Press, 2012), 22.

5 Joseph Keon, *Whitewash: The Disturbing Truth About Cow's Milk and Your Health* (Canada: New Society Publishers, 2010), 191.

6 Paul Solotaroff, "In the Belly of the Beast," *Rolling Stone,* 10 December 2013, http://www.rollingstone.com/feature/belly-beast-meat-factory-farms-animal-activists.

7 Robyn O'Brien, *The Unhealthy Truth: One Mother's Shocking Investigation into the Dangers of America's Food Supply—And What Every Family Can Do to Protect Itself* (New York: Random House, 2009) 99.

8 Robyn O'Brien, *The Unhealthy Truth: One Mother's Shocking Investigation into the Dangers of America's Food Supply—And What Every Family Can Do to Protect Itself* (New York: Random House, 2009), 99.

9 Kurtis Ming, "Call Kurtis Investigates: What's In Your Milk?," CBS Sacramento, 14 May 2012, http://sacramento.cbslocal.com/2012/05/14/call-kurtis-investigates-whats-in-your-milk/.

10 Samuel Epstein, *What's In Your Milk?: An Exposé of Industry and Government Cover-Up on the Dangers of the Genetically Engineered (rBGH) Milk You're Drinking* (Trafford Publishing, 2006).

11 Kathy Murphy, "Business: More Buyers Asking: Got Milk Without Chemicals?" *The New York Times,* 1 August 1999, http://www.nytimes.com/1999/08/01/business/business-more-buyers-asking-got-milk-without-chemicals.html?pagewanted=all&src=pm.

12 Samuel Epstien, "Hormonal Milk and Meat: A Dangerous Public Health Risk," *Huffington Post,* 13 April 2010, http://www.huffingtonpost.com/samuel-s-epstein/hormonal-milk-and-meat-a_b_521932.html.

13 Joseph Keon, *Whitewash: The Disturbing Truth About Cow's Milk and Your Health* (Canada: New Society Publishers, 2010), 62.

14 Suemedha Sood, "Milking It," *The Washington Independent,* published March 25 2008, http://washingtonindependent.com/1882/milking-it.

15 Christine Escobar, "The Tale of rBGH, Milk, Monsanto and the Organic Backlash," *HuffingtonPost,* 3 March 2009, http://www.huffingtonpost.com/christine-escobar/the-tale-of-rbgh-milk-mon_b_170823.html.

16 Joseph Keon, *Whitewash: The Disturbing Truth About Cow's Milk and Your Health* (Canada: New Society Publishers, 2010), 200.

17 Joseph Keon, *Whitewash: The Disturbing Truth About Cow's Milk and Your Health* (Canada: New Society Publishers, 2010), 201.

18 Andrew Martin, "As Recession Deepens, So Does Milk Surplus," *The New York Times,* 1 January 2009, http://www.nytimes.com/2009/01/02/business/02dairy.html?pagewanted=all&_r=0.

19 Joseph Keon, *Whitewash: The Disturbing Truth About Cow's Milk and Your Health* (Canada: New Society Publishers, 2010), 200).

20 Mark Hyman, "Dairy: 6 Reasons You Should Avoid It at All Costs or Why Following the USDA Food Pyramid Guidelines is Bad for Your Health," *Huffington Post,* 1 May 2010, http://www.huffingtonpost.com/dr-mark-hyman/dairy-free-dairy-6-reason_b_558876.html.

21 "Calcium and Milk: What's Best for Your Bone Health," *Harvard School of Public Health,* 2014, http://www.hsph.harvard.edu/nutritionsource/calcium-full-story/.

22 Mark Hyman, Dairy: 6 Reasons You Should Avoid It at All Costs or Why Following the USDA Food Pyramid Guidelines is Bad for Your Health," *Huffington Post,* 1 May 2010, http://www.huffingtonpost.com/dr-mark-hyman/dairy-free-dairy-6-reason_b_558876.html.

23 Joseph Keon, *Whitewash: The Disturbing Truth About Cow's Milk and Your Health* (Canada: New Society Publishers, 2010), 47.

24 "Healthy Eating Plate and Healthy Eating Pyramid," *Harvard School of Public Health,* http://www.hsph.harvard.edu/nutritionsource/healthy-eating-plate/, 4 February 2014.

25 Joseph Keon, *Whitewash: The Disturbing Truth About Cow's Milk and Your Health* (Canada: New Society Publishers, 2010), 31.

26 Joseph Keon, *Whitewash: The Disturbing Truth About Cow's Milk and Your Health* (Canada: New Society Publishers, 2010), 33.

27 Joseph Keon, *Whitewash: The Disturbing Truth About Cow's Milk and Your Health* (Canada: New Society Publishers, 2010), 63.

28 Joseph Keon, *Whitewash: The Disturbing Truth About Cow's Milk and Your Health* (Canada: New Society Publishers, 2010), 58.

29 T. Colin Campbell and Thomas M. Campbell, *The China Study: The Most Comprehensive Study of Nutrition Ever Conducted and the Startling Implications for Diet, Weight Loss, and Long Term Health* (Dallas, TX: BenBella Books, 2004).

30 "Calcium and Milk: What's Best for Your Bone Health," *Harvard School of Public Health,* 2014, http://www.hsph.harvard.edu/nutritionsource/calcium-full-story/.

31 T. Colin Campbell and Thomas M. Campbell, *The China Study: The Most Comprehensive Study of Nutrition Ever Conducted and the Startling Implications for Diet, Weight Loss, and Long Term Health* (Dallas, TX: BenBella Books, 2004).

32 "Calcium and Milk: What's Best for Your Bone Health," *Harvard School of Public Health,* 2014, http://www.hsph.harvard.edu/nutritionsource/calcium-full-story/.

33 "Calcium and Milk: What's Best for Your Bone Health," *Harvard School of Public Health,* 2014, http://www.hsph.harvard.edu/nutritionsource/calcium-full-story/.

34 Joseph Keon, *Whitewash: The Disturbing Truth About Cow's Milk and Your Health* (Canada: New Society Publishers, 2010), 172.

35 "Calcium and Milk: What's Best for Your Bone Health," *Harvard School of Public Health,* 2014, http://www.hsph.harvard.edu/nutritionsource/calcium-full-story/.

Chapter Seven:

1 "USDA Celebrates 150 Years," *United States Department of Agriculture,* 15 April 2014, http://www.usda.gov/wps/portal/usda/usdahome?navid=USDA150.

2 "Mission Statement", *United States Department of Agriculture,* 15 April 2014, http://www.usda.gov/wps/portal/usda/usdahome?navid=MISSION_STATEMENT.

3 Michael Moss, "While Warning About Fat, US Pushes Cheese Sales," *The New York Times,* 6 November 2010, http://www.nytimes.com/2010/11/07/us/07fat.html?pagewanted=all.

4 Rod Leonard, *Losing Control of Food Safety* (Minneapolis, Minnesota: The Institute for Agriculture and Trade Policy, 2007), 2.

5 Rory Freedman and Kim Barnouin, *Skinny Bitch* (Running Press, 2006).

6 Thomas Burton and Martin Fackler, "Mad-Cow Testing on Trial: Should US Start to Screen Every Last Cow as in Japan? A Negligible Cost Increase," *Wall Street Journal,* 2 January 2004.

7 Rory Freedman and Kim Barnouin, *Skinny Bastard: A Kick in the Ass for Real Men Who Want to Stop Being Fat and Start Getting Buff* (Pennsylvania: Running Press, 2009), 157.

8   Rod Leonard, *Losing Control of Food Safety* (Minneapolis, Minnesota: The Institute for Agriculture and Trade Policy, 2007), 1.

9   "FrontLine Modern Meat: Interview Eric Schlosser," *PBS*, http://www. pbs.org/wgbh/pages/frontline/shows/meat/interviews/schlosser.html, 4 February 2014.

10   Elisa Odabashian, "Testimony to the California Legislature on Mad Cow Disease," *Consumers Union*, 24 February 2004.

11   Rod Leonard, *Losing Control of Food Safety* (Minneapolis, Minnesota: The Institute for Agriculture and Trade Policy, 2007), 1.

12   FoxNews "California Company Recalls 87 Million Pounds of Meat," *Associated Press*, 9 February 2014, http://www.foxnews.com/ us/2014/02/09/california-company-recalls-87-million-pounds-meat/.

13   Chris Frates and Shannon Travis, "Unfit for Human Consumption: How Nearly 9 Million Pounds of Bad Meat Escaped into the Food Supply," *CNN*, 2 May 2014, http://eatocracy.cnn.com/2014/05/02/bad-meat-investigation/.

14   Gretchen Goetz, "Who Inspects What? A Food Safety Scramble," *Food Safety News*, 16 December 2010, http://www.foodsafetynews. com/2010/12/who-inspects-what-a-food-safety-scramble/#.UvCqIv-ldWSo.

15   David Wallinga, *Playing Chicken: Avoiding Arsenic in Your Meat* (Minneapolis, Minnesota: The Institute for Agriculture and Trade Policy, 2006), 18.

16   David Wallinga, *Playing Chicken: Avoiding Arsenic in Your Meat* (Minneapolis, Minnesota: The Institute for Agriculture and Trade Policy, 2006), 18.

17   James Andrews, "Poll: Three Quarters of Americans Want More Government Food Safety Oversight," *Food Safety News*, 7 February 2014, http://www.foodsafetynews.com/2014/02/three-quarters-of-amer-icans-want-more-government-food-safety-oversight/#.UvhZrfldWSo.

18 "Examining the Implementation of the Food Safety Modernization Act," *Energy and Commerce Committee,* 5 February 2014, http://energycom-merce.house.gov/hearing/examining-implementation-food-safety-modernization-act#video.

19 Travis Madsen and Benjamin Davis(Frontier Group) and Brad Heavner and John Rumpler, Environment America Research & Policy Center, *Growing Influence: The Political Power of Agribusiness and the Fouling of America's Waterways* (Environment America, 2011).

20 Thomas Stratmann, "Can Special Interests Buy Congressional Votes? Evidence from Financial Services Legislation," American Political Science Association 2002 Annual Meeting, Boston (2002), http://ideas.repec.org.

21 Robbie Feinberg, "Special Interests Heavily Involved in Farm Bill Maneuvering," *OpenSecrets.Org,* 30 January 2014, http://www.opense-crets.org/news/2014/01/special-interests-heavily-involved.html.

22 Travis Madsen and Benjamin Davis(Frontier Group) and Brad Heavner and John Rumpler, Environment America Research & Policy Center, *Growing Influence: The Political Power of Agribusiness and the Fouling of America's Waterways* (Environment America, 2011).

23 Robbie Feinberg, "Special Interests Heavily Involved in Farm Bill Maneuvering," *OpenSecrets.Org,* 30 January 2014, http://www.opense-crets.org/news/2014/01/special-interests-heavily-involved.html.

24 Rigorberto A. Lopez, "Campaign Contributions and Agricultural Subsidies," *Economics and Politics* 13 (3)(2001), 257–78.

25 Robbie Feinberg, "Special Interests Heavily Involved in Farm Bill Maneuvering," *OpenSecrets.Org,* 30 January 2014, http://www.opense-crets.org/news/2014/01/special-interests-heavily-involved.html.

26 Travis Madsen and Benjamin Davis(Frontier Group) and Brad Heavner and John Rumpler, Environment America Research & Policy Center, *Growing Influence: The Political Power of Agribusiness and the Fouling of America's Waterways* (Environment America, 2011).

27 The Johns Hopkins Center for Livable Future, *Feed for Food Producing Animals: A Resource on Ingredients, the Industry, and Regulation,* (Baltimore, Maryland: Bloomberg School of Public Health, 2007), 4–5.

28 The Johns Hopkins Center for A Livable Future, *Feed for Food Producing Animals: A Resource on Ingredients, the Industry, and Regulation,* (Baltimore, Maryland: Bloomberg School of Public Health, 2007), 5.

29 David Robinson Simon, *Meatonomics: How the Rigged Economics of Meat and Dairy Make You Consume Too Much and How to Eat Better, Live Longer, and Spend Smarter* (San Francisco: Conari Press, 2013), 67.

30 Phillip Mattera, *USDA Inc, How Agribusiness Hijacked Regulatory Policy at the US Department of Agriculture* (Washington DC: Organization for Competitive Markets, 2004), 10–11.

31 Robyn O'Brien, The Unhealthy Truth: One Mother's Shocking Investigation into the Dangers of America's Food Supply—and What Every Family Can Do to Protect Itself," (New York: Random House, 2009).

32 Kenneth Vogel, "Obama Administration's Revolving Door," *Politico,* 18 January 2011, http://www.politico.com/news/stories/0111/47713.html.

33 Mark Babineck, "Judge Dismisses Lingering Lawsuit Against Oprah Winfrey," *TexNews,* 18 September 2002, http://www.texnews. com/1998/2002/texas/texas_Judge_dis918.html.

34 David Robinson Simon, *Meatonomics: How the Rigged Economics of Meat and Dairy Make You Consume Too Much and How to Eat Better,* Live Longer, and Spend Smarter (San Francisco: Conari Press, 2013), 53.

35 Brandon Kiem, "Ag-Gag Laws Could Make America Sick," *Wired,* 2 May 2013, http://www.wired.com/wiredscience/2013/05/ag-gag-public-health/.

Chapter Eight:

1 David Robinson Simon, *Meatonomics: How the Rigged Economics of Meat and Dairy Make You Consume Too Much and How to Eat Better, Live Longer, and Spend Smarter* (San Francisco: Conari Press, 2013), xx.

2 David Robinson Simon, *Meatonomics: How the Rigged Economics of Meat and Dairy Make You Consume Too Much and How to Eat Better, Live Longer, and Spend Smarter* (San Francisco: Conari Press, 2013), xxv.

3 David Robinson Simon, *Meatonomics: How the Rigged Economics of Meat and Dairy Make You Consume Too Much and How to Eat Better, Live Longer, and Spend Smarter* (San Francisco: Conari Press, 2013).

4 David Robinson Simon, *Meatonomics: How the Rigged Economics of Meat and Dairy Make You Consume Too Much and How to Eat Better, Live Longer, and Spend Smarter* (San Francisco: Conari Press, 2013), xxi.

5 David Robinson Simon, *Meatonomics: How the Rigged Economics of Meat and Dairy Make You Consume Too Much and How to Eat Better, Live Longer, and Spend Smarter* (San Francisco: Conari Press, 2013).

6 Steven Reinberg, "Almost 10 Percent of US Medical Costs Tied to Obesity," ABC News, 28 July 2009, http://abcnews.go.com/Health/Healthday/story?id=8184975.

7 David Robinson Simon, *Meatonomics: How the Rigged Economics of Meat and Dairy Make You Consume Too Much and How to Eat Better, Live Longer, and Spend Smarter* (San Francisco: Conari Press, 2013).

8 PA Heindenreich, et al, "Forecasting the Future of Cardiovascular Disease in the United States: A Policy Statement from the American Heart Association," *Circulation* 123(8)(2011), 933–944.

9 Union of Concerned Scientists, *The 11 Trillion Dollar Reward: How Simple Dietary Changes Can Save Lives and Money and How We Get There* (2013).

10 Maryn McKenna, "The Biggest FoodBorne Illness Threat May Not Be Addressed By the New Food Safety Law," *Wired,* 28 April 2011, http://www.wired.com/wiredscience/2011/04/foodborne-disease-. threat/?utm_source=Contextly&utm_medium=RelatedLinks&utm_campaign=Previous.

11 *Keeping America's Food Supply Safe* (University of Florida: Emerging Pathogens Institute, 2011).

12 Maryn McKenna, "The Biggest FoodBorne Illness Threat May Not Be Addressed By the New Food Safety Law," *Wired,* April 28 2011, http://www.wired.com/wiredscience/2011/04/foodborne-disease-.threat/?utm_source=Contextly&utm_medium=RelatedLinks&utm_campaign=Previous.

13 Alliance for the Prudent Use of Antibiotics, *The Cost of Antibiotic Resistance to US Families and the Health Care System,* (Tufts University, 2010), http://www.tufts.edu/med/apua/consumers/personal_home_5_1451036133.pdf.

14 Centers for Disease Control, *Antibiotic Resistant Threats in the United States, 2013* (US Department of Health and Human Services, 2013), http://www.cdc.gov/drugresistance/threat-report-2013/pdf/ar-threats-2013-508.pdf.

15 Rachel Zimmerman, "CDC: Millions Acquire Antibiotic-Resistant Infections, Thousands Die Annually," *CommonHealth,* 16 September 2013, http://commonhealth.wbur.org/2013/09/cdc-millions-getting-infections-resistant-to-antibiotics.

16 *Factsheet: Antibiotic Resistance and Animal Agriculture* (Washington DC: Keep Antibiotics Working, April 2010).

17 David Robinson Simon, *Meatonomics: How the Rigged Economics of Meat and Dairy Make You Consume Too Much and How to Eat Better, Live Longer, and Spend Smarter* (San Francisco: Conari Press, 2013), 3.

18 Geoffrey S. Becker, "Federal Farm Promotion (Check Off) Programs," Congressional Research Service Report for Congress (2008), www.nationalaglawcenter.org.

19 David Robinson Simon, *Meatonomics: How the Rigged Economics of Meat and Dairy Make You Consume Too Much and How to Eat Better, Live Longer, and Spend Smarter* (San Francisco: Conari Press, 2013), 7.

20 US Department of Agriculture, "Benefits of Research and Promotion Boards," (2011).

21 *Johanns v. Livestock Mktg Ass'n* (2005) 544 US.550.

22 David Robinson Simon, *Meatonomics: How the Rigged Economics of Meat and Dairy Make You Consume Too Much and How to Eat Better, Live Longer, and Spend Smarter* (San Francisco: Conari Press, 2013), 8.

23 Bill Tomson, "US Makes Special Purchase of $40 Million Chicken Products," *The Wall Street Journal,*15 August 2011, http://online.wsj.com/news/articles/SB10001424053111903392904576510863093422074.

24 Elanor Starmer and Timothy Wise, *Feeding at the Trough: Industrial Livestock Firms Saved $35 Billion From Low Feed Prices* (Global Development and Environment Institute Tufts University, 2007).

25 David Robinson Simon, *Meatonomics: How the Rigged Economics of Meat and Dairy Make You Consume Too Much and How to Eat Better, Live Longer, and Spend Smarter* (San Francisco: Conari Press, 2013).

26 Bryan Walsh, "Getting Real About the High Price of Cheap Food", *TIME,* 21 August 2009, http://content.time.com/time/magazine/article/0,9171,1917726,00.html.

27 David Robinson Simon, *Meatonomics: How the Rigged Economics of Meat and Dairy Make You Consume Too Much and How to Eat Better, Live Longer, and Spend Smarter* (San Francisco: Conari Press, 2013).

28 Pew Commission on Industrial Farm Animal Production, *Putting Meat on the Table: Industrial Farm Animal Production in America* (Maryland: John Hopkins Bloomberg School of Public Health: 2009).

29 Jennifer Sandy, "Factory Farms: A Bad Choice for Rural America," Forum Journal 23 (2009), http://www.preservationnation.org/forum/library/public-articles/factory-farms.html.

30 Emily Main, "Factory Farm Pollution: What You Smell Can Hurt You," *Rodale News,* 21 January 2014, http://www.rodalenews.com/factory-farm-pollution.

31 Doug Gurian-Sherman, *CAFOS Uncovered: The Untold Costs of Confined Animal Feeding Operations* (Cambridge, MA: Union of Concerned Scientists, 2008).

32 Doug Gurian-Sherman, *CAFOS Uncovered: The Untold Costs of Confined Animal Feeding Operations* (Cambridge, MA: Union of Concerned Scientists, 2008).

33 David Robinson Simon, *Meatonomics: How the Rigged Economics of Meat and Dairy Make You Consume Too Much and How to Eat Better, Live Longer, and Spend Smarter* (San Francisco: Conari Press, 2013).

34 Mark Bittman, "Rethinking the Meat-Guzzler," *The New York Times,* 27 January 2008, http://www.nytimes.com/2008/01/27/weekinreview/27bittman.html?ei=5070&em=&en=15ae80659f4ded2b&ex=1202014800&pagewanted=all&_r=0.

35 David Robinson Simon, *Meatonomics: How the Rigged Economics of Meat and Dairy Make You Consume Too Much and How to Eat Better, Live Longer, and Spend Smarter* (San Francisco: Conari Press, 2013).

36 "Obama Signs $1 Trillion Farm Bill Into Law," *Environmental News Service,* 7 February 2014, http://ens-newswire.com/2014/02/07/obama-signs-1-trillion-farm-bill-into-law/.

Chapter Nine:

1 Bryan Walsh, "Getting Real About the High Price of Cheap Food", *TIME,* 21 August 2009, http://content.time.com/time/magazine/article/0,9171,1917726,00.html.

2 Pierre Gerber, Hennin Steinfeld, et al, *Livestock's Long Shadow: Environmental Issues and Options* (Rome: Food and Agricultural Organization of the United Nations, 2007).

3 Bryan Walsh, "The Triple Whopper Environmental Impact of Global Meat Production," *TIME,* 13 December 2013, http://science.time.com/2013/12/16/the-triple-whopper-environmental-impact-of-global-meat-production/.

4 Marla Rose, "The Hunger Shame," *VegNews Magazine,* 87 (Sept-Oct 2012), 40–45.

5   Peter Singer and Jim Mason, *The Ethics of What We Eat: Why Our Food Choices Matter* (United States: Rodale Inc, 2006).

6   Marla Rose, "The Hunger Shame," *VegNews Magazine,* 87 (Sept-Oct 2012), 42.

7   World Hunger Education Service, "2012 World Poverty Facts and Statistics," *Hunger Notes,* Oct. 2012, http://www.worldhunger.org/articles/Learn/world%20hunger%20facts%202002.htm.

8   Pierre Gerber, Hennin Steinfeld, et al, *Livestock's Long Shadow: Environmental Issues and Options* (Rome: Food and Agricultural Organization of the United Nations, 2007).

9   Marla Rose, "The Hunger Shame," *VegNews Magazine,* 87 (Sept-Oct 2012), 42.

10   Pierre Gerber, Hennin Steinfeld, et al, *Livestock's Long Shadow: Environmental Issues and Options* (Rome: Food and Agricultural Organization of the United Nations, 2007).

11   John Robbins, *The Food Revolution: How Your Diet Can Help Save Your Life and Our World* (San Francisco: Conari Press, 2011).

12   Moby and Miyun Park, *Gristle: From Factory Farms to Food Safety-Thinking Twice About the Meat We Eat* (New York: New Press, 2010), 121.

13   Christina Sterbenz and Gus Libin, "7 Charts That Could Convince You to Become Vegetarian," *Business Insider,* 18 October 2013, http://www.businessinsider.com/reasons-to-go-vegetarian-in-charts-2013-10.

14   Pierre Gerber, Hennin Steinfeld, et al, *Livestock's Long Shadow: Environmental Issues and Options* (Rome: Food and Agricultural Organization of the United Nations, 2007).

15   Michael Jacobson, *Six Arguments for a Greener Diet* (Center for Science in the Public Interest, 2006), 93.

16   Pierre Gerber, Hennin Steinfeld, et al, *Livestock's Long Shadow: Environmental Issues and Options* (Rome: Food and Agricultural Organization of the United Nations, 2007).

17   Michael Pollan, "Power Steer," *New York Times,* 31 March 2002.

18   Daniel Imhoff, *The CAFO Reader: Tragedy of Industrial Animal Production* (California: Foundation for Deep Ecology, 2010).

19   Peter Singer and Jim Mason, *The Ethics of What We Eat: Why Our Food Choices Matter* (United States: Rodale Inc, 2006).

20   Daniel Imhoff, *The CAFO Reader: Tragedy of Industrial Animal Production* (California: Foundation for Deep Ecology, 2010).

21   Daniel Imhoff, *The CAFO Reader: Tragedy of Industrial Animal Production* (California: Foundation for Deep Ecology, 2010).

22   Moby and Miyun Park, *Gristle: From Factory Farms to Food Safety-Thinking Twice About the Meat We Eat* (New York: New Press, 2010).

23   Moby and Miyun Park, *Gristle: From Factory Farms to Food Safety-Thinking Twice About the Meat We Eat* (New York: New Press, 2010), 57.

24   Kari Hamerschlag, *The Meat Eater's Guide to Climate Change + Health* (Washington DC: Environmental Working Group, 2011).

25   Kari Hamerschlag, *The Meat Eater's Guide to Climate Change + Health* (Washington DC: Environmental Working Group, 2011), 7.

26   Moby and Miyun Park, *Gristle: From Factory Farms to Food Safety-Thinking Twice About the Meat We Eat* (New York: New Press, 2010), 59.

27   Kari Hamerschlag, *The Meat Eater's Guide to Climate Change + Health* (Washington DC: Environmental Working Group, 2011) 5.

28   Kari Hamerschlag, *The Meat Eater's Guide to Climate Change + Health* (Washington DC: Environmental Working Group, 2011), 3.

29   Kari Hamerschlag, *The Meat Eater's Guide to Climate Change + Health* (Washington DC: Environmental Working Group, 2011), 12.

30   Bryan Walsh, "The Triple Whopper Environmental Impact of Global Meat Production," *TIME,* 13 December, 2013, http://science.time.com/2013/12/16/the-triple-whopper-environmental-impact-of-global-meat-production/.

Chapter Ten:

1   Bryan Walsh, "The Triple Whopper Environmental Impact of Global
     Meat Production," *TIME,* 13 December, 2013, http://science.time.
     com/2013/12/16/the-triple-whopper-environmental-impact-of-global-
     meat-production/.

2   MH Carlsen, BL Halvorsen, K Holte, SK Bohn, S Dragland, et al., "The
     Total Antioxidant Content of More than 3100 Foods, Beverages, Spices,
     Herbs and Supplements Used Worldwide," *Nutr J* 9(2010), 3.

3   Shushana Castle and Amy-Lee Goodman, *Rethink Food: 100+ Doctors
     Can't Be Wrong* (Houston: Two Skirts Productions, 2014), 211–213.

4   Mayuree Rao, Ashkan Afshin, Gitanjali Singh and Dariush Mozaffarian,
     "Do Healthier Foods and Diet Patterns Cost More than Less Healthy
     Options? A Systematic Review and Meta-Analysis," *BMJ Open* 3 (2013),
     January 2014, doi: 10.1136/bmjopen-2013-004277.

5   "Technomic Finds College Students Calling for Healthier Choices and
     Greater Say in Shaping Campus Dining Programs", *PR News Wire*,
     accessed January 2014, http://www.prnewswire.com/news-releases/
     technomic-finds-college-students-calling-for-healthier-choices-and-
     greater-say-in-shaping-campus-dining-programs-127523548.html.

6   "The Real Food Challenge," 5April 2014, http://www.realfoodchallenge.
     org/.

7   "Technomic Finds College Students Calling for Healthier Choices and
     Greater Say in Shaping Campus Dining Programs", *PR News Wire*,
     accessed January 2014, http://www.prnewswire.com/news-releases/
     technomic-finds-college-students-calling-for-healthier-choices-and-
     greater-say-in-shaping-campus-dining-programs-127523548.html.

8   "Fast Food Facts in Brief," *FACTS-Food Advertising to Children and
     Teens at Yale University*, 5 November 2013, http://www.fastfoodmar-
     keting.org/fast_food_facts_in_brief.aspx.

9   Pew Commission on Industrial Farm Animal Production, "Putting Meat
     on the Table: Industrial Farm Animal Production in America," 2008:
     56-95, http://www.ncifap.org/_images/PCIFAPFin.pdf.

INDEX